EVALUATING
NURSING
INTERVENTIONS

To our families, mentors, and colleagues

EVALUATING NURSING INTERVENTIONS
A THEORY-DRIVEN APPROACH

SOURAYA SIDANI
Faculty of Nursing, University of Toronto

CARRIE JO BRADEN
College of Nursing. University of Arizona

SAGE Publications
International Educational and Professional Publisher
Thousand Oaks   London   New Delhi

For information:

SAGE Publications, Inc.
2455 Teller Road
Thousand Oaks, California 91320
E-mail: order@sagepub.com

SAGE Publications Ltd.
6 Bonhill Street
London EC2A 4PU
United Kingdom

SAGE Publications India Pvt. Ltd.
M-32 Market
Greater Kailash I
New Delhi 110 048 India

Printed in the United States of America

Library of Congress Cataloging-in-Publication Data

Sidani, Souraya.
    Evaluating nursing interventions: A theory-driven approach/by Souraya Sidani and Carrie Jo Braden.
        p. cm.
    Includes bibliographical references and index.
    ISBN 0-7619-0315-1 (cloth : acid-free paper).—ISBN 0-7619-0316-X (pbk. : acid-free paper)
        1. Nursing audit. 2. Outcome assessment (Medical care).   I. Braden, Carrie Jo, 1944- .   II. Title.
    RT85.5.S53 1998
    610.73—dc21   97-21227

98 99 00 01 02 03 04   10 9 8 7 6 5 4 3 2 1

Acquiring Editor:	Daniel Ruth
Editorial Assistant:	Anna Howland
Production Editor:	Michele Lingre
Production Assistant:	Karen Wiley
Typesetter/Designer:	Yang-hee Syn Maresca
Cover Designer:	Ravi Balasuriya
Print Buyer:	Anna Chin

CONTENTS

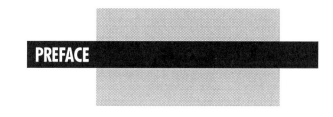

PREFACE

Evaluating the effectiveness of interventions in achieving the desired outcomes is a prerequisite for using interventions in clinical practice. To be able to implement a particular intervention and to use it appropriately in practice, clinicians require knowledge of the specific activities or components of the intervention, their related strength or dosage, the mechanisms underlying the intervention effects, the intervention's intended and unintended effects, the client population that would most benefit from the intervention, and the context in which the intervention is useful. In other words, clinicians need to know which intervention components, at which dosage, under what circumstances, and with which clients, result in which outcomes. This kind of information is essential for expanding the knowledge base for practice and for assisting clinicians in selecting and prescribing the most appropriate intervention to their clients.

Developing this kind of knowledge base for practice necessitates a change in the conceptual analysis and the methodology used in intervention effectiveness research. At the conceptual level, the change has to do with the assumptions underlying clinical effectiveness research. The notion that the intervention will produce the same response in all participants needs to be modified to allow for individual variations in response. Factors other than the intervention that are believed to influence the outcomes of an intervention should be identified a priori and incorporated in a theoretical framework that explains the mechanisms responsible for producing the desired outcomes. At the methodological level, the changes in conducting effectiveness research include judicious use of various types of research design to maximize the validity of the study conclusions when the study is conducted in a clinical setting where multiple extraneous factors have the potential of affecting the intervention outcomes, empirically examining the effects of extraneous factors such as client and setting characteristics on clients' response to treatment, examining the effects of the intervention at the individual or subgroup level, representing the various components of the intervention and the dosage received by the participants as the measure of the independent variable in the data analysis, and using different types of statistical approaches for analyzing the data. In short, the changes are directed toward a more comprehensive approach to effectiveness research for the purpose of developing clinically relevant knowledge that guides practice.

Our contention in this book is that the development of clinically relevant knowledge rests on identifying factors related to the intervention, the intervener, the clients, and the setting that influence the clients' response to the intervention and on determining the impact of these factors on outcome achievement. The identification and analysis of these factors' effects should be guided by the theory underlying the intervention. The intervention theory specifies the nature of the intervention, the nature of the effects expected of the intervention, processes mediating the expected effects, and the conditions under which the intervention processes take place. The intervention theory provides answers to the clinical questions about which intervention would be appropriate for what client population under which circumstances. The intervention theory directs the implementation of the intervention and all aspects of a study aimed at evaluating the effectiveness of the intervention in producing the desired outcomes. It forms the basis for selecting the study design, setting, sample, variables, and measures; for developing the treatment protocol; for formulating and carrying out the data collection procedure; for conducting the analyses; and for interpreting the results, whether favorable or unfavorable. Briefly, the intervention theory provides the rationale for the intervention and dictates research methods. In turn, findings of intervention evaluation research provide feedback for consolidating or refining the intervention. A close link between theory and research is essential for expanding knowledge.

The primary goals of this book are to present a comprehensive and in-depth analysis of the contribution of various factors to the validity of the study findings, to examine how these factors operate, to delineate the role of theory identifying and examining the effects of these factors, and to provide strategies for dealing with these factors successfully. Conventional strategies for dealing with these factors are reviewed and their limitations when used in the field settings are explained. Alternative strategies are suggested. The alternative strategies are geared toward operationalizing the theory-driven approach to effectiveness research that incorporates the conceptual and methodological changes needed for developing clinically relevant knowledge. Expanding clinically relevant knowledge is a means for reducing the gap between research and practice.

The book is intended to expand clinical effectiveness research methods available for investigators. The proposed research methods are most appropriate for evaluating the effectiveness of interventions or programs in practice, that is, under "real-life" conditions; the principles underlying these methods can also be used to guide the initial testing of the intervention efficacy under ideal conditions, however. The content of this book builds on basic intervention/program evaluation topics and addresses advanced issues in detail. The intervention evaluation methods covered in this book should be of interest to graduate students and to junior and senior researchers planning or conducting a study aimed at evaluating interventions. The book content pertinent to the factors that influence the outcomes expected of an intervention could assist investigators conducting meta-analyses examining the effectiveness of a particular intervention and clinicians reviewing or critically appraising the effects of an intervention in preparation for using it in their practice. Whenever possible, examples are provided to illustrate major points of discussion. Readers are strongly encouraged to think of their own work to put the issues discussed in a more familiar context. The book is designed to provide readers with the principles of effectiveness research methodology; we hope that readers will find them useful and will apply them in their own work.

ACKNOWLEDGMENTS

The authors gratefully acknowledge the thoughtful comments and constructive feedback and suggestions offered by Diane Irvine and Lee Sechrest.

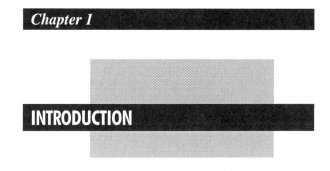

Chapter 1

INTRODUCTION

The social mandate of health-related professions, and in particular nursing, is to provide high-quality care that results in the best health outcomes to clients. Providing and maintaining high-quality care requires the development of a sound knowledge base to enhance the understanding of the clients' clinical condition and guide clinical decision making regarding selecting and implementing the interventions that are most effective in improving the clients' condition. The development and advancement of such clinical knowledge can be achieved through a critical evaluation of health-related interventions. A critical evaluation of interventions consists of determining their effectiveness in producing the desired health outcomes. This chapter presents a brief overview of high-quality care, points to the importance of advancing clinical knowledge, examines the outcomes-focused strategy for evaluating the effectiveness of interventions, and introduces the content to be covered in the remaining chapters of the book.

High-Quality Care: An Overview

The primary concern in health-related and nursing professions is the delivery of services for the purposes of managing presenting problems, preventing untoward conditions, and promoting proper functioning and well-being. To be successful in achieving these goals, professional health services should be of high quality. High-quality care can be broadly defined as the delivery of care that results in the best health outcomes for clients. Redfern and Norman (1990) characterized health care services that are accessible, acceptable, efficient, effective, and appropriate, as high quality. Accessible services are readily available and can be used by clients when needed. Acceptable services are agreeable to potential clients. Efficient services are worth their cost; they are capable of producing the expected results within the specified time frame and the limits of available resources. Effective services are those that achieve the intended benefits for the clients. Appropriate services are those that meet the actual needs of the clients or resolve their presenting problems.

The emphasis on providing and maintaining high-quality care has been dictated by professional regulatory bodies, health care consumers, health care insurance and coverage agencies, and society at large. Professional regulatory bodies develop, review, and improve standards of care. They ensure that clinicians follow the established standards in their everyday practice. Standards of care reflect the ideal practice, that is, what the professionals should do to provide services of high quality (Redfern & Norman, 1990). Standards of care are developed by experts in the field, based on empirical research. They are used as guides to clinical practice and as criteria for evaluating the performance of clinicians. With the expansion in health knowledge and technologies and the dissemination of health-related information to the public, consumers have been demanding increasing accountability on the part of professionals. Accountability is defined as the obligation of professionals to clients to provide high-quality care with predictable outcomes. Thus, consumers are asking that the care they receive is effective in resolving their problems and appropriate in meeting their individual needs. Health care and government agencies, as well as third-party payers, are demanding increased financial accountability, holding professionals responsible for delivering cost-effective high-quality care.

Evaluating the quality of care provided to clients is a necessity that stems from the social contract between health professionals and society. Implicit in this social contract is the accountability of health professionals to clients for the safety of the services they offer and for the provision of care with predictable outcomes.

Requirements for Maintaining High-Quality Care

High-quality care refers to the delivery of health-related services that are appropriate, efficient, and effective, resulting in the best outcomes for the clients. This definition implies that to provide quality care professionals are required to apply knowledge in such a way as to benefit the clients' health (Donabedian, 1980). To benefit the clients' health, the care planned and implemented by professionals should be based on an adequate understanding of the clients' problems, the mechanisms through which the health care services or interventions resolve the identified problem, and the outcomes expected as a result of the implementation of the intervention. Inadequate knowledge in any of these areas jeopardizes the safety and the quality of health care, with the potential for untoward effects.

Clinicians need to have a clear understanding of the clients' problem requiring resolution. They need to be aware of its causative factors in order to design and implement interventions that are effective in treating it. If the same problem is related to different causative processes, then different interventions are required to resolve it. For instance, dyspnea may be precipitated by either psychological or physiological factors. The psychological status of increased situational anxiety stimulates the sympathetic nervous system, which results in rapid, shallow breathing and subsequent perception of dyspnea (Altose, Cherniack, & Fishman, 1985). Physiological changes such as airway obstruction prevent adequate ventilation and consequently lead to shallow breathing that is perceived as dyspnea (Gottfried, Altose, Kelsen, & Cherniack, 1981). The type of intervention that can be used to relieve dyspnea depends on the causative factors of the condition. Listening to music is effective in reducing anxiety and consequently dyspnea; therefore, it is most appropriate when anxiety is the precipitating factor. Conversely, performing deep-breathing exercises or pursed-lip breathing is effective in relieving dyspnea associated with airway obstruction. Although the two types of intervention are used to resolve the same clinical problem and have the same ultimate outcome, the mechanisms mediating their effects differ. Each is appropriate in a particular situation and is characterized by distinct causative processes underlying its effects.

In addition to knowledge of the causative processes underlying the clinical problem and the effects of the intervention, clinicians require a clear understanding of the specific nature of the intervention. Clinicians need to know the activities that constitute the intervention and the details of how to carry them out. They also need to know how the intervention works in producing the expected outcomes. The following aspects of implementing an intervention should be made explicit for the clinician: what activities it comprises and how and when to perform each activity, at what level, with which intensity, and for how long. In the above example, listening to music relieves dyspnea. A clinician who plans to prescribe it to a client must know the following: (a) the method for delivering the music (Is the client to listen to music as background music or through earphones?), (b) the kind of music most effective in relieving dyspnea (Is it soft, relaxing, or rhythmic music?), (c) the activity the client should be doing while listening to music (Which activity would be most effective: lying down, sitting in a chair, standing, or performing activities of daily living?), (d) the appropriate time for listening to music (Does the client listen to music before experiencing dyspnea, i.e., prophylactically, or as soon as he or she experiences difficulty breathing?), (e) the length of time the client has to listen to music to get relief (Does the client listen to music for 5, 10, 20, 60 minutes or longer?), (f) the frequency with which the client has to listen to music (How many times a day? a week?), and (g) how music relieves dyspnea (What are the processes or mechanisms through which music alleviates dyspnea?).

Knowledge of the causative processes underlying the clinical problem and of the effects and the nature of the intervention are essential to but not sufficient for providing high-quality care. From a clinical perspective, the care offered should be also acceptable and appropriate to the individual clients. Care that is tailored to the particular needs of clients is considered high-quality care. Thus, clinicians should be able to discern the clients that would most benefit from a particular intervention. They should also be able to identify the conditions under which the intervention would be most effective and the type of and extent to which modifications in the way the intervention is implemented would be admissible, that is, resulting in the same health outcomes expected of the intervention. The complexity of the clinical phenomena and of the clinical setting often requires some adaptation and flexibility in delivering the intervention. In the example about shortness of breath, some clients may like to listen to music if the music is played in the background, if they listen to music while sitting in their recliner, and if the music is "classical." In contrast, others may prefer to listen to "new age" or "easy-listening" music, through earphones, and while carrying out their daily activities.

In summary, providing high-quality care requires in-depth knowledge of (a) the nature of the presenting clinical problem that is to be treated, including its causative factors; (b) the nature of the intervention to be used for treating the problem, including the processes underlying the effects of the intervention, the activities to be performed and the frequency, duration, and intensity of these activities that are needed to produce the desired effects; (c) the outcomes expected as a result of implementing the intervention; and (d) the contextual and individual-client factors that affect the delivery of the intervention and its underlying mechanisms (Chen, 1990; Lipsey, 1993). From a clinical perspective, clinicians must know which specific component of the intervention, with what strength, under what conditions, results in which outcomes, for which clients. This kind of knowledge allows them to plan and deliver care that is effective, efficient, and appropriate, meeting the individual needs of clients—that is, high-quality care.

Evaluating the Quality of Care

The interest in providing, monitoring, and evaluating the quality of health care led to the development of many health care quality models. These models guided the understanding of what constitutes high-quality care and proposed strategies for evaluating or improving the quality of care (Deming, 1986; Donabedian, 1988; Donabedian, Wheeler, & Wyszewianski, 1982; Larrabee, 1996). Of these, Donabedian's model gained acceptance among a variety of health professionals (Mitchell, 1993). The model proposes that high-quality care depends on three essential elements: structure, process, and outcome. *Structure* refers to the prerequisites and resources used in the provision of care to clients. Structure covers factors related to the physical and organizational work environment and to the technical and professional characteristics of the care providers. *Process* refers to the services offered to clients, including the actual activity performed by health care providers and the decision making underlying its implementation. *Outcomes* reflect the end results of care; they represent the changes observed in the clients' health condition.

Examining the quality of care consists of comparing the characteristics of the work environment and the services or care provided against acceptable standards (Candeias, 1991) and determining their effectiveness in achieving the intended benefits. Earlier efforts to evaluate the quality of health care focused on examining the structure and processes of care. For instance, the majority of research projects conducted in the last three decades of the 20th century focused on the characteristics of nursing personnel; the supply, organization, and distribution of nursing services; nurses' job satisfaction; and some nursing care issues such as infection control that would enhance care quality (Burns & Grove, 1993). Currently, evaluating the quality of care focuses on examining outcomes achievement.

Outcomes-Focused Evaluation

Client outcomes are considered the yardstick, or the standards, for assessing the efficiency and effectiveness of health services (Bond & Thomas, 1991; Kremer, 1991). The assumption underlying the use of outcomes as standards of care is that "variations in clinical practice are associated with differences in patient outcomes and resource use" (Raskin & Maklan, 1991, p. 164). Therefore, the health outcomes achieved by clients are viewed as indicators of the quality of the care they received. Monitoring outcome achievement (e.g., by comparing the clients' status to critical pathways) is viewed as an acceptable, cost-efficient, and patient-centered method for evaluating the quality of the care given. The Joint Commission on Accreditation of Hospitals Organization encourages the use of outcomes as criteria guiding quality assurance audits. The Agency for Health Care Policy and Research has launched a new program of research, the Medical Treatment Effectiveness Program. Patient outcomes research teams were designed to examine variability in outcomes in particular clinical conditions, such as hip fracture, cataract, and heart disease; to identify sources of variability associated with the care provided; and to determine the most effective and cost-effective intervention for producing the desired outcomes. The objective of these efforts was to assist clients, payers, and providers to "make rational medical care-related choices based on a better insight into the effectiveness of these choices on the patient's life" (Slater, 1991, p.131). The ultimate goal is to properly and effectively manage the care to improve its outcomes.

The increasing interest in patient outcomes is a function of the inter-action among sociopolitical and economic factors. The provision of spe-cialized and sophisticated health care services resulted in increased health care costs. The increased health care costs prompted government officials and public administrators to question the performance and productivity of health professionals and organizations, demanding greater attention to the efficiency and effectiveness of health care services, and to reduce expen-diture while maintaining quality. Cost-containment strategies led health care professionals to offer high-quality services at lower prices within a highly competitive environment and to measure the impact of these serv-ices on clients' health status, thus demonstrating the accountability of their professions to clients and to society. Enlightened health care consumers are demanding not only greater accountability from all segments of the health care field but also informed participation in decision making regard-ing their care. Informed decision making requires that the consumers be aware of health care options available to them and, more important, of the consequences of each option. Briefly, the general concern with maximiz-ing the quality of health care within the limits of scarce resources per-suaded health professionals of the necessity to examine the effectiveness of the services or the interventions they provide in achieving desired patient outcomes (Griffiths, 1995; Hegyvary, 1991, 1993; Jennings, 1991; Jones, 1993; Parker, 1983; Peters, 1988; Shonkoff, Hause-Cram, Krauss, & Upshur, 1988).

Evaluation Methods

The concern with evaluating the quality of care led to a critical evaluation of the effectiveness of health services in producing the desired outcomes. Health services consist of diverse and multiple interventions that professionals perform on behalf of their clients in order to achieve desirable changes in the clients' status. Evaluating the quality of health services can be done at two levels of analysis: general, or macro; and specific, or micro, levels. At the macro level, the emphasis is on evaluating the quality of the overall care services delivered to clients during a particular episode of care. Hospital quality assurance programs illustrate the macro level of quality evaluation. At the micro level, the emphasis is on evaluating the quality of particular programs or interventions; this usually entails examining their effectiveness in producing expected outcomes. Although both levels of analysis are valuable and needed, this book focuses on evaluating particular interventions or programs. The effectiveness of interventions or programs is receiving increasing attention among health professionals as they are held accountable for the care they provide (Snyder, Egan, & Najima, 1996). Knowledge of which particular intervention to use, for which clients, to produce which outcomes forms the basis for providing high-quality care (Moritz, 1995).

Interventions refer to treatments, therapies, procedures, or actions implemented by health professionals to and with clients, in a particular situation, to move the clients' condition toward desired health outcomes that are beneficial to the clients (Jennings,1991; McCloskey et al., 1990; Moritz, 1995; Snyder et al., 1996). Specific interventions are directed toward the alleviation of particular or well-defined clinical problems; they address one aspect or dimension of health. Examples of specific interventions are preoperative instructions, perinatal coaching, range of motion exercises, and breathing and coughing exercises. Programs incorporate a combination of specific interventions that address various dimensions of the clients' health and that are given together, as a package, with the aim of improving their overall health condition. Examples of health programs are (a) cardiac rehabilitation programs involving different interventions such as counseling, stress management techniques, smoking cessation, exercise training, and dietary management; and (b) the Preparedness, Enrichment, and Predictability (PREP) home health care program composed of expanded in-home services for frail elder people, an advice line providing advice and reassurance as well as linkage with other health care services, and a keeping-in-touch system in which the health status of clients is monitored continuously (Archbold et al., 1995). It is important to clarify that in some situations the interventions target the health care providers or the setting in which health care is provided, such as continuing education programs, institution of total quality management programs, and changing the staffing pattern on a unit. Although the target of this type of intervention differs from that of health-related interventions of primary interest in this book, the strategies and methods for evaluating both kinds of interventions are similar.

The critical evaluation of interventions or programs consists of the application of a systematic process for the purpose of determining whether or not the interventions or programs are effective in achieving their intended effects. Usually, evaluating the effects of interventions is programmatic. Initially, the intervention effects are examined under controlled conditions that permit the manipulation of the treatment and the control of extraneous factors, so that changes in the outcomes can be directly linked to the intervention. Once it is demonstrated that the intervention produces the expected effects under controlled conditions, the ability of the intervention to achieve the same outcomes in the field or natural setting is examined. Field testing is conducted to assess the outcomes of an intervention as it would actually be applied in the "real world." The term *field* refers to any setting in which the intervention is delivered, such as a hospital unit, nursing home, school, community center, or the client's home. Evaluating the effectiveness of interventions in field settings (hereafter called effectiveness research) provides information regarding the impact of interventions on outcomes, which is useful to distinguish effective, efficient, and appropriate interventions from ineffective, inefficient, and inappropriate ones. The primary concern in effectiveness research is to demonstrate that the changes in the intended outcomes observed in the clients after the implementation of the intervention are directly linked to the intervention itself and not to other factors that may be present under field conditions and may influence outcomes achievement. In more traditional terms, the concern is in determining the causal relation between the intervention and the intended outcomes, meaning that the intervention did, indeed, cause or result in the observed outcomes.

The research strategy most commonly advocated and often used in effectiveness research is the true experimental design. The true experimental design is characterized by random assignment of participants to the experimental groups, control of contextual or situational factors that may potentially confound the participants' response to the treatment, and manipulation of the treatment (i.e., giving it to all participants in the experimental group in the same way and at the same level and withholding it from participants in the control group). This experimental control reduces the potential effects of confounding factors. Therefore, it increases the confidence in attributing the observed changes in the outcomes to the intervention being evaluated. As a result, the validity of the inference about the effectiveness of the intervention is enhanced (Cook & Campbell, 1979).

The focus on assessing outcomes as indicators of the effectiveness of interventions or programs reinforces the use of the traditional experimental design in effectiveness research. Random assignment of participants to the experimental and control groups enhances the distribution of uncontrollable factors across the groups, thereby reducing the potential influence of the factors on the achievement of the intended effects. Consequently, the net impact of the intervention on the outcomes can be determined. The findings of outcomes-focused, experimental endeavors provide valid empirical evidence supporting the claim that the intervention does produce the desired changes in the clients' health condition. Thus, the causal link between the intervention and the intended outcomes is established under well-controlled conditions, thereby answering, with confidence, the question, Is the intervention effective in producing the intended outcomes?

Weaknesses of Outcomes-Focused Evaluation

Focusing only on client outcomes to determine the effectiveness of interventions or programs has been criticized at the theoretical, empirical, and clinical levels.

Theoretically, the term *outcomes* refers to the results or the consequences of care, that is, to the measurable changes in the clients' health condition reflecting the intended responses to an intervention. Outcomes have the advantage of being comprehensive and reflective of what preceded them. Outcomes are affected not only by the intervention delivered but also by a host of factors related to the clients, to the humanistic or interpersonal aspect of care, and to the setting or environment in which care is provided. Clinical reality shows that outcomes vary regardless of the intervention delivered. There are situations in which the clients' health condition improves even if the intervention is not implemented, and there are situations in which the clients' health condition deteriorates even if the most effective and appropriate intervention is implemented (Brooten & Naylor, 1995; Hegyvary, 1991; Taylor, 1974). Therefore, focusing on the assessment of outcomes alone provides an incomplete and inaccurate picture of the impact of a particular intervention. Outcomes alone do not tell precisely what may have caused the favorable or unfavorable intervention effects (Bloch, 1975; Peters, 1988; Strupp, 1996).

Empirically, outcomes-focused evaluation provides a narrow and sometimes distorted understanding of the effects of the intervention delivered (Chen & Rossi, 1989). Focusing on the examination of outcomes alone (a) falls short of assessing and analyzing the mechanisms linking the intervention to its effects; and (b) does not take into consideration the potential influence of extraneous factors on the specified outcomes, such as the clinically acknowledged influence of client characteristics on the response to treatment. When the causative mechanisms underlying the intervention effects are not assessed, failure of the intervention in producing the expected outcomes can not be clearly explained, since the failure could be due to either the intervention having a poor conceptual framework or the intervention being improperly implemented (Chen & Rossi, 1989; Goldfried & Wolfe, 1996; Lipsey, 1993). When the influences of extraneous factors are not examined, the conditions strengthening or weakening the intervention effects cannot be determined (Costner, 1989).

Clinically, evaluating the intervention using the traditional experimental design falls short of providing specific information to guide practice. Results of an effectiveness study usually indicate that the intervention is or is not effective in producing some outcomes, while holding extraneous confounding factors constant. But the causal inferences regarding the intervention effectiveness are not necessarily relevant to the natural, real-life situation of everyday practice. In real-life situations, multiple factors interact in a complex network of causes and effects. Thus, the effects of an intervention tested under experimental control may not appear due to the interference of the naturally occurring extraneous factors (Newman & Tejeda, 1996). An understanding of the interrelations among these factors and of their effects on the intervention and its expected outcomes is important. Clinicians require detailed knowledge of how an intervention works, at what optimal dosage, with which client population, under what conditions, to produce which outcomes. This detailed information is needed in order to prescribe the intervention correctly and apply it successfully in everyday practice (Goldfried & Wolfe, 1996; Marfo & Dinero, 1993).

Organization of the Book

There is no single methodology that is most appropriate for conducting intervention effectiveness research, but several strategies are presented in this book. The premises on which this book is based are the following (a) Although the focus on clients' outcomes may be legitimate to determine the effectiveness of interventions, studying outcomes independent of the processes underlying the intervention and of significant extraneous factors is inadequate for developing clinically relevant knowledge. (b) The rigor of true experimental designs is essential for ruling out alternative explanations of the observed effects and for enhancing the validity of inferences regarding the intervention effectiveness. But their results are of limited generalizability or applicability to practice; to promote the applicability of the findings to the clinical setting, the designs of effectiveness studies should be representative of clinical situations. (c) An accurate and valid evaluation of the effectiveness of the intervention cannot be accomplished without a clear understanding of the theoretical framework underlying its effects; this understanding of the why and how of an intervention permits its application in a responsive fashion and its adaptation to varying circumstances encountered in clinical practice (Lipsey, 1993).

The thesis advanced in this book is that intervention effectiveness research should be theory driven in order to develop and expand clinically relevant knowledge. The theory underlying the intervention needs to be explicitly stated and tested. The intervention theory specifies the nature of the intervention, the nature of the effects expected of the intervention, the processes mediating the expected effects, and the conditions under which the mediating processes occur. Thus, the intervention theory identifies factors other than the intervention that could influence outcome achievement and guides the analyses of their impact on outcomes. These factors are related to the clients receiving the intervention, to the health care professionals delivering the intervention, to the conditions under which or the setting in which the intervention is provided, to the nature of the intervention and the integrity of its implementation, and to the selection of outcome variables that reflect the intended treatment effects.

The overall goal of this book is to present strategies for operationalizing the theory-driven approach to effectiveness research. The specific purposes of this book are to critically analyze the nature of factors that could influence the effectiveness of an intervention in producing the desired outcomes, to examine their impact on the validity of the study conclusions, to determine the role of theory in examining these factors, and to discuss strategies for dealing with them. The proposed methods are appropriate for studies evaluating the effectiveness of interventions and programs as applied in field, or real-life, settings, under less controlled conditions. The principles underlying these methods can also be used to guide the initial testing of intervention efficacy under controlled conditions and the planning and organizing of critical appraisal of the literature and meta-analytic studies that aim at determining the effectiveness of particular interventions.

This book is organized around the factors that could influence the effectiveness of intervention outcomes and that are addressed by the intervention theory. Chapter 2 describes the methodology of the traditional approach for examining the outcomes of health and nursing interventions and reviews its strengths and weaknesses. The weaknesses of this traditional approach are discussed for cases in which the study findings are significant or nonsignificant. The theory-driven approach is presented as an alternative approach for evaluating outcomes of interventions. In Chapter 3, the theory-driven approach to effectiveness research is described and illustrated. Chapter 4 focuses on the nature and influence of factors related to the clients on the effectiveness of intervention. Client-related factors influence the effects of interventions on the outcomes by increasing inter-individual differences in the response to treatment. Strategies for dealing with these extraneous sources of variability in outcomes are discussed. In Chapter 5, the role of the intervener and setting-related factors on intervention effectiveness are examined. These factors influence the delivery of the interventions and the participants' response to treatment. Methods for dealing with them are explored. Chapter 6 underscores the importance of measuring process factors. Process factors relate to aspects of the intervention, its implementation, and the mechanisms underlying its effects. Variability in the delivery of the intervention results in variability in the intervention strength received by individuals and consequently in variability in outcome achievement. Methods for representing the intervention and the mechanisms mediating its effects and for monitoring its implementation are presented. Chapter 7 emphasizes the importance of selecting outcome variables that are sensitive to the intervention being studied and outcome measures that are reliable, valid, and sensitive to change. Methods for ensuring and examining the properties of measures selected to operationalize outcome variables are described. The final chapter summarizes the implications of the theory-driven approach to effectiveness research. Examples from published research and from the Self-Help Intervention Project (SHIP) study will be used to illustrate the points of discussion throughout the book. The next section presents an overview of the SHIP study.

Overview of the
Illustrative Study

The SHIP study (Braden, Mishel, Longman, & Burns, 1989) was funded by the National Cancer Institute (RO1 CA48450) for the purposes of evaluating the effectiveness of three interventions in promoting self-care, psychosocial adjustment, and life quality in breast cancer patients receiving adjuvant medical therapy. The three intervention approaches were a self-help course, an independent study self-help course, and a telephone delivered uncertainty management intervention. The SHIP interventions were informed by two complementary middle-range nursing theories: learned response to chronic illness (Braden, 1990) and uncertainty in illness (Mishel, 1988; 1990).

According to the theory of learned response to chronic illness, learning is initiated upon diagnosis of a disease condition with the perceived *severity of illness* serving as the stimulus for learning. Entrance into the chronic illness learning frame also results in exposure to adversities, such as *uncertainty* about the illness, that undermine initiation of *enabling skills* (problem solving, cognitive reframing, and belief in self). The adversities can be mediated relative to achievement of desired goals such as having *confidence* in one's level of *knowledge, self-care,* and *self-help.* When one has confidence in knowing about management of the illness and finds ways of continuing valued adult role activities (self-help) and of instituting strategies to manage disease- or therapy-related symptoms (self-care), one's *life quality* is maintained or enhanced.

According to the theory of uncertainty in illness, *uncertainty* is generated when symptoms and treatment-related events occur without pattern, are unfamiliar (lack *event familiarity*) or differ from past experience or expectation (lack *event congruence*). The ability of the individual to accurately perceive these events is influenced by the individual's information-processing capacity. Accurate perception of events is increased when there is *trust* and confidence *in the health care provider* and the existence of a *social support* structure that encourages communication about the illness experience. Uncertainty is perceived as a neutral experience until it is appraised as either a danger (*threat appraisal*), indicating the experience of uncertainty is threatening, or as an opportunity (*challenge appraisal*), indicating the uncertainty is a desirable experience. When uncertainty is appraised as a danger, actions are directed at *managing uncertainty* to limit its negative impact on psychological adjustment. When uncertainty is appraised as an opportunity, actions are directed at *maintaining uncertainty* to influence *psychosocial adjustment.* The SHIP intervention activities based on the learned response to chronic illness theory focus on enhancing enabling skills, and the intervention activities based on the uncertainty in illness theory focus on uncertainty management directed to conservation of enabling skills. The self-help course activities focus on enhancing the enabling skills of problem solving, cognitive reframing, and belief in self. They were delivered in a series of six 90-minute classes, offered once a week for 6 weeks. A standardized teacher guide included the amount of time allotted to each activity. Six different teachers (four nurses, a social worker, and a counselor) led the classes over the 3 years of enrollment in the interventions. All teachers participated in a teacher training program. Two teachers shared the responsibility for each class to increase attention to class participants' interactions and processing needs while maintaining adherence to the teaching protocol.

The independent study self-help course was based on the activities used in the self-help course. The learning activities were formatted into six lessons and enclosed in a loose-leaf notebook. The notebook was designed to facilitate and direct independent study.

The uncertainty management intervention consisted of a telephone contact with a nurse having a background in oncology and mental health. The nurse initiated the contact at least once a week for 6 weeks. Women were invited to call the nurse manager any time during the 6-week period. The exchanges with the women were guided by a standardized assessment/appraisal/intervention protocol. The protocol served as a basis for (a) identification of new areas of uncertainty, (b) selection of the intervention to resolve the uncertainty, and (c) reassessment of areas of uncertainty and determination of resolved uncertainties. The uncertainty interventions were organized around five goals: (a) strengthening an existing cognitive structure and reinforcing opportunity appraisals, (b) promoting cognitive structure formation, (c) reducing negative certainty used in instances when a perception of certain negative outcome was inappropriate or incorrect, (d) regulating emotional response, and (e) managing continual uncertainty. All nurses participated in training prior to providing the interventions.

Table 1.1 Outcomes of the SHIP Effectiveness Study

Interventions	*Outcomes*
Uncertainty management	Improved management of uncertainty
Self-help course	Reduced uncertainty
Combined	Enhanced enabling skills
Independent study	Increased knowledge
	Improved self-care
	Improved self-help
	Enhanced psychological adjustment
	Enhanced life quality

Combination self-help course/uncertainty management and independent study self-help/uncertainty management were essentially participation in two interventions during the same 6-week time period.

The expected outcomes of the SHIP interventions included (see Table 1.1) (a) management of uncertainty (use of strategies to limits its impact), (b) enabling skills (problem solving, cognitive reframing, and belief in self), (c) self-care (the level of role behaviors devoted to enhancing or maintaining health), (d) self-help (the perceived level of involvement in carrying out adult role activities), (e) psychological adjustment (the positive or negative emotional mood experienced at a certain point in time), (f) knowledge (the level of knowledge related to cancer and its treatment and to strategies for managing one's condition), (g) quality of life (the level of overall satisfaction with life), and (h) uncertainty (a cognitive state of lack of form or structure to the events, i.e., ambiguity, occurring in a specific illness condition). Data were collected at six points in time: baseline (T1), timed to be after the adjuvant medical treatment protocol was under way to allow for the emergence of treatment-related side effects; T2, 6 to 8 weeks following T1; T3, 3 months following T2; T4, 6 months after T2; T5, 9 months after T2; and T6, 1 year after T2. *The findings from the SHIP study reported here for illustration relate to the subgroup of 56 women with complete data across the six points of measurement.*

Summary

Evaluating the effectiveness of nursing interventions and programs in producing the desired outcomes when delivered in the field setting is a necessity. It is essential for developing and expanding clinically relevant knowledge to assist clinicians in selecting and prescribing the most appropriate interventions to their clients. Such knowledge provides clinicians with a clear understanding of the clients' presenting problem, the mechanism through which the intervention resolves the problem, the outcomes expected as a result of the intervention, and the conditions under which the intervention is most effective. The application of such knowledge in practice enhances professional accountability and the quality of care. Using the true experimental design with a focus on assessing outcomes only as indicators of the intervention effectiveness has some limitations in achieving clinically relevant knowledge (Hegyvary, 1991; Moritz, 1995). The theory-driven approach to intervention evaluation is proposed as an alternative methodology for conducting clinical effectiveness research. The theory-driven approach guides the examination of factors that could influence outcome achievement and that are of primary interest for the proper application of the intervention in the field setting. This book discusses the theory-driven approach to effectiveness research and presents strategies for operationalizing it.

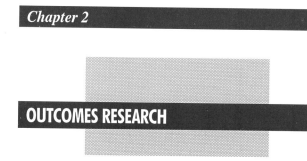

Chapter 2

OUTCOMES RESEARCH

Outcomes research refers to studies focusing on assessing the consequences of an intervention or program. Knowledge of which intervention is effective in producing desired outcomes assists clinicians in judging the value of various treatment modalities, in selecting appropriate interventions that best meet the clients' needs, and in using scarce resources efficiently (Ellwood, 1988; Mariner, 1994; Moritz, 1995). Development of outcomes-related knowledge requires a systematic approach to evaluating intervention effectiveness in achieving the desired changes. The conventional true experimental design is considered the standard approach for intervention effectiveness research. This chapter describes this conventional approach. Its strengths and limitations are discussed. The theory-driven approach to evaluation is introduced as a strategy to overcome the limitations of the conventional approach.

Evaluating the effectiveness of an intervention or program can be programmatic and sequential. First, the intervention is examined under ideal, controlled conditions using the conventional experimental design. This is essential to determine the extent to which the intervention is effective in producing the intended effects. The well-controlled setting is conducive to the creation of the ideal conditions under which the intervention is expected to work. The ideal conditions require substantial restrictions in context and variations in treatment implementation. These restrictions are accomplished through conducting the experiment in the same setting and in the same context across all subjects and through standardizing the treatment, that is, giving it in the same way, in the same amount, and by the same trained intervener, to all subjects. Once the initial efficacy of the intervention is established, the intervention effects are examined under field conditions, that is, in the actual or natural setting in which the intervention will be ultimately applied (i.e., clinical trials) (Newman & Tejeda, 1996). Some interventions do not lend themselves to this kind of programmatic testing. Rather, they require initial testing in the field, under real-life conditions. Evaluating the effectiveness of a particular intervention that is delivered to clients under real-life conditions is challenging. The real or natural setting in which the intervention is applied is complex and does not lend itself to control of factors that may influence the intervention effects. Multiple factors in the field or natural setting interfere with the ability to carry a true experimental study, with the delivery of the intervention as planned, and with the clients' response to treatment. The alternative research methodology needed to meet this challenging evaluation task is presented in this book.

The Conventional Approach

In this section, the conventional approach for effectiveness research is described; its strengths and limitations when used in effectiveness research are discussed.

Background

The conventional approach to effectiveness research refers to the use of the true experimental design for evaluating the effectiveness of an intervention in producing the expected outcomes. It is outcomes focused in that it aims at determining whether the intervention "works" or "does not work," that is, whether it achieves the desired outcomes (Moritz, 1995). To claim that the intervention does, indeed, produce the expected outcomes, researchers have to demonstrate a causal connection between the treatment and the outcomes (Cook, 1993). Please note that the terms *intervention* and *treatment* are used interchangeably.

In an intervention effectiveness study, the causal connection between the intervention and the expected outcomes is demonstrated if the following criteria for causality are met:

1. Temporal order: The expected changes in the clients' condition follow—and do not precede—the delivery of the intervention; otherwise, the observed changes are attributed to factors other than the intervention, since they occurred irrespective of the treatment implementation.
2. Covariation: The expected effects tend to occur in the presence or with the delivery of the intervention and tend not to occur in its absence or when it is not implemented.
3. Contiguity: The application or manipulation of the treatment results relatively soon in a change in the effects. It is difficult to infer causality when the changes in outcomes do not appear immediately after the treatment implementation, because a series of other events or factors could mediate the causal effect of the intervention on the outcomes during the elapsed period of time.
4. Congruity: The observed changes are consistent and congruent with the nature and strength of the intervention; that is, drastic changes in an outcome usually cannot be attributed to a weak treatment and the outcomes affected should be meaningfully related to the nature of the intervention.
5. Ruling out all other plausible causes of the effects: The observed changes in the outcomes are validly attributed to the intervention and not to alternative factors present in the situation studied (Einhorn & Hogarth, 1986). In Cook and Campbell's (1979) terms, threats to the internal validity of the study findings are eliminated as plausible explanations of the observed outcomes.

Meeting the criteria for causality requires the investigator to manipulate the delivery of the treatment, to control extraneous factors that could influence the intervention effects, and to measure the outcomes before and after the implementation of the treatment. The conventional approach to effectiveness research facilitates the accomplishments of these requirements, as will be described in the next section.

Strengths of the Conventional Approach

The strengths of the conventional approach to effectiveness research lie in its features that permit the demonstration of the causal connection between the intervention and the outcomes. The experimental design allows the investigator to control various aspects of the experimental condition so as to maximize variability in the outcomes attributed to the presumed cause and to minimize extraneous sources of variation that could present threats to the study validity. The true experimental design is most appropriate in establishing all the criteria for causality.

In this design, the experimenter manipulates the intervention. Manipulation entails giving the treatment to a subgroup of subjects and withholding it from another. The treatment is administered under the control of the experimenter in terms of timing, content, and method of delivery. Therefore, in the experimental design, the treatment precedes the effects, thus meeting the temporal order criterion. In addition, the experimenter measures the outcomes before and after implementation of the treatment. Measuring the outcomes immediately after the delivery of the treatment ensures that treatment and effects are adjacent in time and space, thus meeting the contiguity criterion.

Covariation and congruity are established by examining differences in (a) the level on the outcomes measured at posttest, between the subjects who received the treatment and those who did not: and (b) the level on the outcomes between the pretest and posttest, measured on subjects who received the treatment. The treatment is claimed to be effective if a statistically significant difference in the outcomes is observed between the means of the experimental and control groups or if a significant difference in the mean level of the outcomes is observed between pretest and posttest in the experimental group.

The true experimental design is appropriate for ruling out alternative plausible causes of the observed effects. The experimenter carefully selects the subjects according to a set of inclusion and exclusion criteria. The purpose of subject selection is to create a sample that is more or less homogeneous on some characteristics thought to be correlated with the outcomes or to have the potential of moderating the subjects' responses to the treatment. This initial subject variability, if not controlled for through random assignment of subjects to the experimental groups, threatens the validity of the causal claim regarding the effectiveness of the treatment in producing the desired outcomes. In an experimental study conducted in a laboratory setting, the researcher can also control factors in the environment that could affect the treatment outcomes. The investigator controls this extraneous source of variance by ensuring that all subjects are tested under the same experimental conditions, thus rendering the effects of the extraneous factors constant.

Incorporating a control group in which subjects do not receive the treatment is another feature of the true experimental design necessary for ruling out alternative explanations of the observed effects. The control group is used for comparative purposes: If the same changes are observed in subjects assigned to the experimental and the control groups, then the changes cannot be caused by the treatment. Rather, they are attributed to other extraneous factors occurring in both groups simultaneously (Cook & Campbell, 1979).

In summary, the conventional true experimental design is considered the most appropriate in achieving the goal of outcomes-focused effectiveness research, that of claiming that the treatment is effective in producing the expected outcomes. The characteristic features of the true experimental design, namely, random assignment, manipulation, and control, provide the researcher with mechanisms that minimize the potential threats to the validity of the causal connection between the treatment and its effects. But despite its advantages, the conventional approach may be difficult to apply when evaluating interventions in the field or natural setting.

Difficulties in Using the Conventional Approach in the Field

The strengths of the conventional true experimental design in maintaining internal validity and consequently the validity of the causal connection between the intervention and the expected outcomes prompted researchers to use it when evaluating the effects of interventions in the field. The field setting is complex, involving multiple factors that are interrelated, that influence the outcomes expected of interventions, and that cannot be controlled by the investigator. Therefore, the field setting presents difficulties in carrying out experiments.

In field experiments, the researchers conduct their study in collaboration with the staff members employed in the setting in which the intervention is being tested (such as the hospital unit or the community center) . The researchers require the assistance of staff members in recruiting potential subjects and sometimes in delivering the intervention. However, staff members may interfere with the research activities. They may present inaccurate information of the study to potential participants or they may be selective in recruiting clients. For instance, they can recruit clients who would most benefit from the intervention, resulting in selection bias, which is a threat to the validity of the study conclusions. Staff members may defeat random assignment of clients to the experimental and control group, because of ethical and emotional dilemmas associated with denying the intervention to clients who need it and because of their professional obligation to provide suitable treatments to meet the clients' needs (Devine, Wright, & Joyner, 1994). Staff members can resist the idea of randomization because it contradicts the principles of clinical decision making as to which clients would benefit from the intervention. When staff members are aware of the randomization process, such as knowing what would be the group assignment of the next subject selected, they can defer referring a client to the study until the client's assignment coincides with the experimental group (Lam, Hartwell, & Jekel, 1994). Improper randomization may break down the equivalence of the treatment and the control groups on some characteristics related to the outcomes, which threatens the validity of the causal connection between the treatment and its effects (Cook & Campbell, 1979; Devine et al., 1994). Furthermore, if staff members interfere with randomization by communicating or providing the experimental intervention to all participants, the experimental and control groups become equal in terms of the treatment received, thus invalidating any comparisons between the groups (Cook & Campbell, 1979; Stevens, 1994). Finally, staff members can "bad-mouth" the idea of random assignment by exaggerating the differences between the experimental and control conditions when recruiting clients for the study. In doing so, they violate the neutral presentation of the different interventions and set the clients up for a win-lose situation, leading to subject demoralization in the group receiving the less desirable treatment (Schumacher et al., 1994).

Demoralization threatens the validity of a study findings. First, demoralized clients may retaliate by responding or performing very poorly, creating a potential for an overestimation of the treatment effects and making it wrong to attribute the posttest differences between the groups to the treatment. Second, clients receiving the less desirable treatment may drop out of the study. Attrition reduces the sample size and consequently the statistical power to detect significant effects. Also, attrition presents a threat to the validity of conclusions, since those who dropped out may differ on some characteristics from those who stayed. Last, clients who received the less desirable treatment may become resentful and attempt to compensate for their resentment by seeking alternative, favorable treatments, thus making it very difficult to detect any significant difference between the groups (Cook & Campbell, 1979; Schumacher et al., 1994). In addition to interfering with the random assignment of subjects to the experimental and control groups, staff members can influence the implementation of the intervention. When several staff members are involved in implementing the intervention at different occasions and in different clinical sites, as in a multisite clinical trial, the actual intervention delivered may vary. Staff members may have to adapt the prescribed intervention activities to fit the demands of the situation they are in or their individual characteristics may affect the mode of delivering the intervention or the nature of their interaction with clients. The end result of this variability in implementing the intervention is variance in the outcomes achieved by the participants that cannot be attributed to the treatment. Therefore, the ability to demonstrate the causal connection between the intervention and outcomes is weakened. These challenges become more prominent when the study is conducted in a primary care setting, in which the participants themselves are in control of the intervention implementation (Donner, 1992). For instance, when clients are instructed to perform exercises at home, the type and intensity of the exercises performed by each client can deviate from what is expected and vary among participants.

Finally, it is difficult to control all aspects of the field setting, especially in a primary care setting, that influence the delivery of the intervention or its effects. For instance, the relaxing effects of soft music are weakened if the subjects listen to background music in a hospital unit characterized by disturbing noise, uncomfortably low ambient temperature, and frequent interruptions. These characteristics of the clinical setting cannot be controlled by the investigator. They vary across sites and consequently across participants, introducing extraneous variability that weakens the causal intervention-outcomes relation.

Various strategies have been proposed to improve the randomization procedure and treatment implementation in field experiments. Examples of strategies to improve randomization include explaining the purpose and method of randomization to staff members, pointing to the advantage of randomization in resolving ethical and emotional dilemmas in situations in which resources are scarce (Devine et al., 1994), incorporating input from staff members in the design of the field experiment, gathering data on staff and clients' reaction to randomization and examining its influence on outcomes (Orwin, Cordray, & Huebner, 1994), not involving staff members in the randomization procedure (e.g., staff members can be requested to refer interested clients to the research staff, who strictly follow the randomization procedure), using alternative designs that do not require randomization such as the delayed-treatment design or the multiple-baseline design (Schumacher et al., 1994). Providing comprehensive training to interveners, and monitoring the delivery of the experimental intervention as well as the treatments received by clients in the control group are examples of strategies to enhance treatment implementation.

Diverse retention strategies have been suggested and used to minimize subject attrition from the experimental and control groups. Examples of retention strategies are maintaining good rapport and communication with referring staff, centers, or agencies, as well as participants in the study; personalizing the relationship with and demonstrating a "caring attitude" to participants, such as sending them holiday cards; providing tangible rewards to participants, such as reimbursement for transportation (McNeely & Clements, 1994); making research involvement convenient and rewarding for participants by attending to their preferences, for example in the location and method of data collection; and maintaining some form of regular contact with participants if the study is longitudinal (Ribisl et al., 1996).

Although these strategies improve the conduct of field experiments and ultimately enhance their validity, true experimental designs used in outcomes-focused effectiveness research have some limitations in developing the clinically relevant knowledge needed for providing high-quality care.

Limitations of the Conventional Approach

The conventional, outcomes-focused approach to effectiveness research produces results indicating that if the treatment is made to vary, by giving it to one group and withholding it from the other, while holding constant all other factors that might influence the outcomes, the effect or outcome varies with the treatment and would not have varied had the treatment not been present (Cook, 1993). These findings, however, do not provide for any causal explanation of the observed effects, are not necessarily generalizable to the clinical setting, and do not account for differential response to the intervention. Consequently, they do not contribute to the development of the clinical knowledge needed for providing high-quality care, as described in the first chapter.

In the next sections, the limitations of the conventional approach to effectiveness research are discussed. The limitations relate to the weaknesses of the conventional approach in providing for causal explanations of what went on, to the restricted generalizability of findings, and to the focus on statistical rather than clinical significance of findings.

Limitation 1: Causal Explanation

The outcomes-focused, experimental approach to effectiveness research increases the validity of the connection between the intervention and the outcomes but does not provide for causal explanations.

It is important to note that some effectiveness studies are guided by a theoretical framework that explains the linkages between the intervention and its intended outcomes. Nonetheless, the variables mediating the interventions effects, although mentioned at the theoretical level, are not measured and their mediating effects are rarely tested empirically. Rather, they are assumed to have taken place if a significant intervention impact on the outcomes is detected.

The outcomes-focused, experimental approach to effectiveness research is primarily concerned with demonstrating that the intervention produces the desired outcomes. It is less interested in providing causal explanations of the observed effects. Causal explanations identify *how* or *why* a causal connection occurs. They specify (a) the mechanisms underlying the effects of the treatment that represent the chain of events or changes that link the treatment to the expected outcomes, and (b) the conditions under which the effects of the treatment occur (Cook, 1993). Hence, causal explanations are needed to account for significant and nonsignificant findings. When the findings are statistically significant, causal explanations delineate how the intervention "works" or how the favorable outcomes were obtained. When the findings are not statistically significant, knowledge of how the intervention is supposed to work assists in identifying the nature and location of the deficiencies, or "what went wrong" (Chen, 1990). The limitations of the conventional approach in providing for causal explanations are discussed next.

Table 2.1 Weaknesses of Outcomes Research

A. When findings are significant
 1. Not representing and empirically testing the causal mechanisms underlying treatment effects
 2. Underrepresentation of multidimensional interventions
 3. Lack of attendance to multiple causes explaining the outcomes
 4. Uniformity assumptions
 5. Limited generalizability and clinical applicability of findings

B. When findings are not significant
 1. Lack of understanding of "what went wrong"
 2. Inability to rule in or out threats to statistical conclusions and internal and construct validity
 3. Inability to rule in or out poor treatment conceptualization or implementation

---

Weaknesses of the Conventional Approach When the Findings Are Significant

The weaknesses of outcomes-focused research lie in the lack of adequate representation and empirical examination of the causal mechanisms underlying the intervention effects and consequent limited generalizability and clinical applicability of the findings (see Table 2.1). Outcomes research uses the conventional experimental design in which the intervention or program is administered, as a whole package, to the subjects, and the outcome variables are measured at least once prior to and once after implementation of the treatment. This approach to evaluating the effects of a treatment has been labeled the black box approach, since observed variations in the outcomes are attributed to the treatment, regardless of what actually happened between the implementation of the treatment and the appearance of the effects. The interventions become like "buttons that, when pressed, produce useful effects" (Lipsey, 1993, p.8).

This approach reflects a simple cause-effect, reductionistic, and linear view of phenomena, which is inconsistent with clinical reality, in which multiplicity of causes and complexity of human phenomena are the norms. The multidimensionality of health and illness requires the application of complex treatment modalities that often address the various domains of health. For instance, cardiac rehabilitation is offered as a comprehensive program of interventions that aid patients in adjusting to their illness and the required medical regimen. These interventions include prescriptions of physical exercises, dietary instructions for weight control and blood lipid reduction, instructions on taking medications, stopping smoking, and modifying responses to stress (Miller, Wikoff, Garrett, McMahon, & Smith, 1990). Evaluating the effectiveness of this program as a single packaged treatment underrepresents its multidimensionality, oversimplifies its complexity, and makes it difficult to explain the processes that are triggered by its implementation and that are responsible for the favorable changes.

Thus, it is impossible to recognize (a) what are the key variables or events mediating the program's effects, (b) which component of the program is critical in achieving which outcomes, (c) what level of the treatment is necessary for the program to be effective in producing the desired outcomes, (d) under what condition(s) and for which group of clients the treatment is most effective, and (e) when the outcomes are expected to take place. Oldridge, Guyatt, Fischer, and Rimm (1988) and Bittner and Oberman (1993) reviewed the results of randomized clinical trials of cardiac rehabilitation programs involving exercise and risk management. The pooled results indicated reduced cardiovascular mortality. Despite the overall benefit of cardiac rehabilitation, the authors did question the mechanisms by which exercise and risk management reduce mortality. This example illustrates the importance of examining not only the end results of a program but also its components and the mechanisms responsible for producing these effects. Oldridge et al. (1988) wondered whether the provision of information and training in cardiac rehabilitation or the circumstances under which it is provided resulted in the observed benefit.

Focusing only on the effects of an intervention or program, without consideration of its complexity and multidimensionality and without understanding and empirically examining the processes underlying its effects, is not informative. When the process underlying the intervention effects is not examined, one cannot know what exactly caused the favorable outcomes, especially when dealing with complex systems of human beings characterized by a network of multiple causes, multiple effects, and mutual causation (Hegyvary, 1993). The lack of attendance to multiple causes of an intervention's outcomes is another weakness of experimental, outcomes-focused approach. Although the results of a study may show that an intervention has a positive impact on patients, many scholars realize that in real-life situations a multitude of factors contribute to the outcomes of any intervention (Marfo & Dinero, 1993). Patients' outcomes are influenced not only by the intervention provided but by many other factors, such as the restorative processes inherent in each individual, the environmental conditions under which the intervention is administered, the social condition of the patients, demographic factors, and the interpersonal and the technical performance of the intervener during treatment delivery (Barlow, 1996; Bond & Thomas, 1991; Hollon, 1996; Jones, 1993; Lohr, 1988; Strupp, 1996). The lack of concern for identifying and determining the influence of these factors in the experimental, outcomes-focused approach to effectiveness research is related to the experimental control exerted over these factors and to the uniformity assumptions underlying the experimental design. Controlling for these factors is achieved by making them constant across subjects (e.g., giving the treatment under the same conditions and selecting subjects based on well-defined inclusion and exclusion criteria to reduce the sample heterogeneity), thereby nullifying their impact on the causal intervention-outcomes link. The uniformity assumptions state that the subjects enter the treatment with the same characteristics, that the intervention is delivered in the same way to all participants, and that the treatment produces the same response across subjects. These assumptions detract from examining differential subjects' responses to treatment associated with the various factors operating in the clinical setting. Knowledge of how, when, for whom, and under what conditions the intervention works is a prerequisite for the generalizability of its effects (Lipsey, 1993), for improving or refining the intervention (Chen & Rossi, 1980), and for its clinical applicability. Such documentation guides clinicians' decision making about which intervention to provide, to what type of clients, and under what conditions.

To illustrate the weaknesses of the conventional approach to effectiveness research when the findings are significant, let us take the example of an educational intervention provided to cardiac patients admitted to a step-down unit. The intervention consists of three group sessions covering content related to symptoms that may be experienced as a result of the disease process; to strategies for preventing or managing these symptoms such as diet, exercise, and stress-reduction behaviors and techniques; and to pharmacologic regimen. Results of the effectiveness study show that the patients gain some disease and treatment-related knowledge and have improved functional status. But the results did not determine (a) if state anxiety experienced by patients during hospitalization has any influence on their ability to gain knowledge; (b) if the timing of the sessions is optimal (i.e., whether patients benefit most if the instructions are given before or after discharge); (c) if and to what extent the severity of illness affects the patients' functional status and how the intervention helps given this situation; (d) if and to what extent the drug therapy plays a role in producing the favorable outcomes; and (e) if the delivery of the intervention requires special interpersonal skills or expertise on the part of the intervener and therefore whether it can be given by staff nurses working on the step-down unit. Answers to these questions are needed to support the claim that the educational intervention is effective and can be offered to all cardiac patients by the staff nurses caring for them, to achieve the desired outcomes.

In summary, the outcomes-focused experimental approach to effectiveness research has the following limitations when the findings are significant: (a) simplistic representation of the treatment (as experimental vs. control group) resulting in inadequate understanding of how multicomponent interventions or programs work in field settings; and (b) focus on input and output only with a lack of attendance to multiple causes for the observed outcomes, resulting in limited generalizability and clinical applicability of the intervention.

Weaknesses of the Conventional Approach When the Findings Are Not Significant

The weaknesses of the outcomes-focused experimental approach to effectiveness research are more prominent when the findings are not significant (see Table 2.1). When the findings are not significant, researchers cannot accurately identify what went wrong, or the nature and location of the deficiencies. The primary question here is, Was the treatment or the research method defective? The researchers must embark on a tedious journey in search of potential threats to validity. First, researchers may blame the statistical aspects of the study for the failure to detect significant findings. Low statistical power related to a small sample, violated assumptions of statistical tests, and unreliability of the outcome measures are likely to be considered first. If ruled out as potential factors responsible for the observed nonsignificant findings, the researchers address subjects' selection and heterogeneity. The influence of subjects' characteristics, or initial nonequivalence despite randomization, is examined. An analysis of covariance is done to partial out this source of extraneous variability in the outcomes. If the findings are still not significant, threats to internal validity (history, maturation, testing, instrumentation, mortality, diffusion or imitation of the treatment, compensatory

equalization of treatment, compensatory rivalry, and resentful demoralization) are considered and ruled in or out as potential sources for the
deficiencies, based on an analytical exercise undertaken by the researchers.
Next, the following threats to construct validity are examined: hypothesis
guessing, evaluation apprehension, mono-operation and monomethod bias,
experimenter expectancies, inadequate preoperational explication of constructs, confounding constructs, and interaction of different treatments (for
a description of these threats to validity, refer to Cook & Campbell, 1979).
Intervention failure is considered next. Failure is associated with either
inadequate implementation or poor conceptualization of the treatment or
both. Inadequate implementation refers to issues of intervention delivery.
The questions addressed here are, Was the intervention given at all? Was
the intervention given as planned? (Boruch & Gomez, 1977) Was the
amount of the intervention sufficient to produce the desired effects? Poor
conceptualization of the intervention is often thought of as the reason for
treatment failure after ruling out inadequate implementation. Poor conceptualization refers to invalid theoretical underpinnings of the intervention
and to invalidity of the intervention in the target client population. The
primary question addressed here is, Is the intervention, as conceptualized,
expected to produce the specified effects? The issue at hand involves the
validity of the mechanisms mediating the effects of the treatment and the
validity of the prediction that the treatment affects the outcomes examined.
Therefore, evaluating the conceptualization of the intervention requires a
meticulous examination of the chain of events linking the intervention with
the expected outcomes, reanalyzing the plausibility and the logical sequence of the events in relation to alternative explanations of why and how
the treatment works, and determining if the hypothesized sequence of
mediating mechanisms did occur.

Let us take the example of the educational intervention for cardiac
patients on the step-down unit to illustrate the weaknesses of the conventional approach to effectiveness research when the findings are not significant. In this example, the likelihood of intervention failure resulting from
inadequate implementation is relatively high. The educational group sessions are not delivered to all patients assigned to the experimental group
simultaneously, due to logistical reasons: Patients are admitted to the unit
at different points in time and different sessions are offered at different
periods in order to reach as many patients as needed. Therefore, the
sessions may not be given in exactly the same way to all experimental

subjects. Furthermore, the dynamics of the group sessions may be modified due to possible differences in the characteristics of the groups or to the improved skills, over time, of the intervener running the group sessions. In addition, subjects may not be able to attend all three sessions as planned or they may not be able to sit through a whole session; thus, they receive only part of the intervention. These factors result in variability in the treatment implementation, leading to variability in outcomes achievement among the participants and consequently to nonsignificant findings. Poor conceptualization of the intervention is illustrated by a nonsignificant effect of the educational intervention on perceived life satisfaction. Satisfaction with life is operationally defined as the perceived discrepancy between aspiration and achievement (Campbell, Converse, & Rodgers, 1976). As defined, life satisfaction is relatively stable and seems less susceptible to change related to external and objective situation, since people appear to be successful in modifying their aspirations to accommodate changes in their health condition (Campbell, 1981). Therefore, expecting that attending three group sessions will have a direct positive impact on patients' life satisfaction, in a short period of time, does not seem plausible, realistic, or defensible. Rather, the effect of the educational intervention on life satisfaction, if any, seems to be indirect, mediated through improved symptoms management and functional and emotional status.

In summary, researchers attempting to explain nonsignificant findings in effectiveness research should attend to three possible sources of failure: (a) the research method, involving all potential threats to the study validity, including statistical conclusions, internal construct validity; (b) the treatment implementation, that is, the actual delivery of the intervention; and (c) the conceptual underpinnings of the treatment, that is, the plausibility of the causal links between the intervention and the outcomes. Outcomes-focused effectiveness research, relying on the black box approach, does not provide for evaluating the implementation and conceptual underpinnings of the treatment. The intervention is viewed as a package delivered in a standard form to all experimental subjects. Furthermore, researchers evaluate the end results of the packaged intervention, irrespective of the mechanisms mediating the expected effects. In fact, most outcomes research has been based on simple linear main effect models of intervention (Hegyvary, 1993; Moritz, 1995; Shonkoff et al., 1988). Consequently, the factors identified as contributing to or accounting for the nonsignificant findings in outcomes research cannot be ruled in as threats to validity. Their identification remains as the best guess of what went wrong; that is, the black box approach to outcomes research does not provide for explanations of nonsignificant findings or for empirical evidence supporting them.

Limitation 2: External Validity

The outcomes-focused, experimental approach to effectiveness research produces results that are not necessarily externally valid or generalizable to other client populations, treatments, and settings.

The experimental design is considered the gold standard for establishing the causal connection between the intervention and outcomes. Randomization, manipulation, and control of extraneous factors are the characteristic features of true experimental designs that enhance internal validity (Cook & Campbell, 1979; Jacobson & Christensen, 1996). It is exactly these features, however, in addition to sample selection, that make the experimental designs vulnerable with respect to external validity, or reproducibility of the findings across subjects, settings, and intervention implementation procedures such as modification of the intervention activities and dosage (Barlow, 1996; Conrad & Conrad, 1994; Cronbach, 1992; Seligman, 1996).

Practical considerations often limit the sample size of randomized studies. To compensate for small samples, subjects are selected on the basis of strictly defined inclusion and exclusion criteria that ensure that all cases are suitable candidates for the treatment and that ensure reasonable homogeneity within groups. Ensuring within-groups homogeneity reduces variability among subjects on the intervention outcomes that is not attributable to the intervention. Variability in outcomes could be associated with extraneous factors, such as some subjects' characteristics, with the potential of influencing the response to the intervention. For example, severity of illness is a subjects' characteristic that has a direct impact on the outcome of improved functional status; if severity of illness is not controlled for, it results in differences in posttest functional status that cannot be attributed to the intervention being evaluated. Minimizing within-groups homogeneity reduces the error term in statistical testing, which increases the likelihood of detecting significant intervention effects

(Lipsey, 1990; Schwartz & Fox, 1995). Nonetheless, these significant effects may not generalize to other clients encountered in everyday practice, who may experience the same clinical problem treatable with the intervention along with some of the exclusion criteria. Furthermore, the strict eligibility criteria restrict the study sample to a small proportion of the population and consequently the sample size is relatively small. Small samples may not be representative of the target population. For example, Close, Burkey, Kazak, Danz, and Lange (1995) conducted a clinical trial to examine the effects of chemotherapy infusion at home on the clinical and psychological status of children with cancer. During the 5 years of the study period, the investigators were able to recruit only 14 families, representing about 20% of eligible subjects. Subjects were excluded if both parents were working or the mother was occupied with other young children at home and for psychological ineligibility. But the excluded subjects represent a large proportion of the target population.

In addition to restrictions in sample selection, participants' self-selection is another feature of true experiments that limits the external validity of their findings. Participants' self-selection is associated with some patients' and trials' characteristics. Findings of different trials point to various factors influencing the patients' decision to participate in a clinical trial. These factors can be categorized into patients' characteristics and the intervention's characteristics. Generally, subjects' demographics and health characteristics affect their decision to participate. Participants in clinical trials tend to be women, of older age, of higher income groups, of the dominant ethnic group, unemployed, with fewer social resources, disabled, with low functional status, sicker, or with an internal orientation to locus of control. It is difficult to recruit individuals of minority and socio-economically disadvantaged groups (for details, refer to Pletsch, Howe, & Tenney, 1995). Patients' participation is also influenced by their attitudes, including wanting to get the best care possible, trusting the health care professionals and the hospital involved in the study, believing that participation would help "fight the illness," judging that the benefits of participation outweigh the risks, and thinking that the condition would get worse without treatment. In contrast, patients' refusal to participate in a trial is related to feelings of being experimented on, fears of toxicity, transportation problems, preference for another treatment, patient relocation, lack of interest in the study, being busy, and being "too sick" (Kotwall, Mahoney, Myers, & Decoste, 1992; Schwartz & Fox, 1995). The intervention characteristic that is frequently reported as playing a major role in the decision to participate is the perceived attractiveness of the experimental and control conditions. Patients tend to refuse participation if the conditions are perceived to be of unequal attractiveness. Concern about the potential of adverse effects from the experimental treatment is another reason for refusal to participate (Schwartz & Fox, 1995). Clients who agree to participate in an experimental study may differ significantly on various personal and medical characteristics from those who are eligible but decline participation. These differences result in selection bias, which, in turn, may limit the generalizability of the findings, in that the findings may not be applicable to members of the target population who declined participation due to particular characteristics.

The issue of external validity extends to other aspects of the experiment. The random assignment procedure is unrepresentative of actual clinical practice in which clients are given the most appropriate treatment as judged by the clinician, based on their identified problems and needs. Random assignment is an atypical method that clinicians would rarely, if ever, use. Clinicians want to know who would benefit most from the intervention and which client characteristic(s) would potentiate or weaken the effects of the intervention. Therefore, random assignment is of no use as a procedure for deciding who gets the intervention in a real-life situation (Conrad & Conrad, 1994). There is an increasing demand to examine the role of individual characteristics in shaping the intervention effects, that is, in enhancing or impeding outcomes achievement. Knowing who can best benefit from a service is critical for improving the efficient use of available resources (Bauman, Viadro, & Tsui, 1994; Daro & McCurdy, 1994; Marfo & Dinero, 1993; Newman & Tejeda, 1996). Random assignment controls for the personal characteristics that might result in differential intervention effects.

In addition to random assignment, the setting and the method for delivering the intervention in an experimental study may limit its transferability to the clinical setting. The intervention is usually designed and implemented under the researcher's control. The interveners are selected on the basis of well-defined professional characteristics (i.e., qualifications and skills) that are needed for a successful implementation of the intervention. These characteristics influence the intervention delivery, potentially leading to experimenter bias and consequent inability to reproduce the effects of the intervention in everyday practice.

Like the subjects in a study, program staff are also aware of their participation in the study and may alter the treatment or control it in subtle ways,
in reaction to the research. [For example,] people delivering a new experimental treatment would be more excited about the treatment and motivated
to prove that it works or the researcher may have chosen program personnel who have special training, skill, and interest that will not be so readily
available when the treatment is attempted at other sites. (Conrad & Conrad,
1994, pp. 12-13)

Interveners participating in randomized studies use protocols that are to be
followed throughout the study. These protocols may require some modifications or adaptations to fit the practice setting, may require skills and
abilities and a level of judgment that may not be readily available to the
typical practitioner, and may require conditions or equipment that are not
available in some clinical settings (Droitcour & Chelimsky, 1995). The
effects of an intervention evaluated under these ideal conditions may not
be observed under field conditions in which clinicians may not be well
trained in applying the intervention, may not possess all the skills needed
for delivering it, or may have to modify slightly the intervention protocol
to fit with the demands of the clinical situation at hand. Furthermore, the
control of the experimental condition and of the subjects' inclusion and
exclusion criteria limits the reproducibility of the intervention effects in
actual practice. For instance, in real-life conditions, patients do not necessarily meet all the inclusion and exclusion criteria as discussed earlier and
they may be receiving other treatments in conjunction with the intervention
being evaluated (the additional treatments could have constituted the
exclusion criteria). Interaction of the intervention with other treatments is
possible and alters the evaluated intervention effectiveness (Conrad &
Conrad, 1994).

In summary, the characteristics of the subjects, interveners, and setting
are factors that influence treatment delivery, potentially confounding its
effects. Consequently, the reproducibility, or generalizability of the expected intervention effects to day-to-day practice, is jeopardized (Goldfried & Wolfe, 1996).

Limitation 3: Clinical Significance

*The outcomes-focused, experimental approach to effectiveness re-
search determines the statistical but not the clinical significance of the
intervention effects.*

Traditionally, the effects of the intervention are examined by comparing the mean level on the outcomes achieved by the experimental and control groups after treatment delivery. A statistically significant difference between the groups' means indicates that the observed difference is reliable rather than questionable and is beyond what would have been expected by chance alone (LeFort, 1993). Experiments are inherently designed to demonstrate that the observed intervention effects are statistically significant.

Experimenters can manipulate various aspects of the study design to increase the likelihood of detecting statistically significant effects, such as increasing the number of subjects, altering the significance level chosen, and using lengthy measures of variables to reduce measurement error. These manipulations, however, limit the usefulness and applicability of the findings in clinical settings (LeFort, 1993; Scheinder & Darcy, 1984). Also, experiments and their associated statistical testing are concerned with differences at the group level, based on the uniformity assumption that all patients exhibit the same response to the intervention—that is, the intervention has homogeneous effects (Marfo & Dinero, 1993). Although this uniformity assumption facilitates data analysis in effectiveness research, it is inconsistent with clinical reality. Statistical tests "provide no information on the variability of response to treatment within the sample; yet information regarding within-treatment variability of outcome is of the utmost importance to clinicians" (Jacobson & Truax, 1991, p. 13).

From a clinical perspective, patients experiencing the same health problem have different needs that require delivery of interventions on an individualized basis. Patients also differ in ways that demand some modification of the intervention or of its mode of delivery. Furthermore, the same intervention is not expected to have a uniform impact across patients. The patients' response is rather idiosyncratic where variations in the level and trajectory of change in the outcomes are expected. Conducting the statistical analyses at the group level, as is usually done in effectiveness research, is congruent with the uniformity assumption. Individual responses are treated as error deviations when, in fact, they should be examined carefully, as they form the basis for clinical practice, in which differences in the type and degree of outcomes are normative among patients (Howard, Moras, Brill, Martinovich, & Lutz, 1996; Jennings, 1991).

In summary, findings of the outcomes-focused, experimental approach to effectiveness research do not provide sufficient information for clinicians to determine whether a particular intervention is helpful for specific clients. What is needed for conducting intervention effectiveness research are strategies that maintain the rigor of the true experimental designs in ruling out alternative explanations and achieving valid inferences about the intervention effects; yet the strategies should be representative of clinical situations in order to enhance the transferability and applicability of the findings to the clinical setting, and they should be conducive to the development of knowledge that would guide clinical practice.

The Alternative: Theory-Driven Approach

Outcomes evaluation falls short of empirically examining the mechanisms explaining the relationships between the intervention and the expected outcomes and does not take into consideration variability in the implementation of the treatment and the potential influence of extraneous variables on both the treatment implementation and on the specified outcomes. Therefore, the validity of outcomes research findings is questionable, which limits their usefulness and makes difficult their application in the field or natural setting. To be valid, informative, and useful in guiding practice, clinicians, who represent the primary consumers of research findings, need to (a) have a clear understanding of the role of context variables in determining the effectiveness of an intervention in producing the desired outcomes (*context variables* refer to extraneous factors such as social, environmental, setting, and individual or personal factors that could influence the implementation and the outcomes expected of the intervention) (Finney & Moos, 1989; Heller, 1990; Jones, 1993; Shonkoff et al., 1988), (b) have an adequate knowledge of the processes underlying the intervention effects, (c) have a clear specification of the intervention in terms of identifying its components and their related dosage (Chen & Rossi, 1989; Marfo & Dinero, 1993; Scott & Sechrest, 1989), (d) identify outcomes that are sensitive to the intervention (Chen & Rossi, 1987; Griffiths, 1995; Lipsey, 1990; Stewart & Archbold, 1992, 1993), and (e) specify which outcomes are most pertinent to particular client populations (Marfo & Dinero, 1993). In short, there is a call to "progress beyond simply relating variables [intervention and outcomes] toward analyzing multiple dimensions of factors and intervening conditions that lead to the outcomes" (Hegyvary, 1993, p. 150). In other words, there is a call to determine *which interventions, with which dosage, under what circumstances, and with which clients, result in which outcomes.*

This kind of information is essential for developing and expanding the knowledge base for clinical practice and for assisting clinicians in selecting and prescribing the most appropriate intervention to their clients. Providing the appropriate intervention, at the right dose, to produce the outcomes desired for the clients, defines quality of care.

It is evident that the conventional approach to effectiveness research does not lend to the development of the practice-oriented knowledge described above. Consequently, what is needed to improve the validity of outcomes research and to enhance the applicability of its findings in practice is a theory that attempts to explain "what goes on" in a particular situation. In effectiveness research, the theory provides for a comprehensive understanding of the intervention effects, including the nature of the intervention, the causal processes underlying its effects, the magnitude and timing of the anticipated changes, and the conditions under which it is successful. The specificity of the knowledge provided by an intervention theory guides the design of effectiveness research studies; assists in the interpretation of findings, whether significant or nonsignificant; and guides the application of findings in clinical practice. A theory specifies the how, why, when, where, for whom, and for what purpose for a treatment. Clinicians need this specific information to prescribe the interventions in "a responsive fashion rather than in mechanical or stereotyped form. When the 'why' and the 'cause' are known, an approach can be adapted to varying circumstances" (Lipsey, 1993, p. 9), thus meeting the needs of particular client groups. Therefore, theory-based effectiveness research is a useful strategy for testing the processes underlying the intervention effects, for identifying the conditions under which the intervention is most effective, for building clinically relevant knowledge, and consequently for reducing the gap between research and practice.

Summary

The conventional strategies focusing on outcomes expected of interventions and controlling for extraneous factors that might influence the expected outcomes fall short of representing the real world and of maintaining the clinical relevance of findings. Hegyvary and Chamings (1975) acknowledged the drawback of outcomes-focused research in examining the complexity of clinical reality:

It is obvious that we cannot look at complex situations involving human beings, machines, fears, personal motives, timetables, and all the pressures of the hospital environment with simplistic ideas of cause and effect. To say that one variable is the cause of a favorable . . . outcome is to express lack of understanding of the patient care system. Patient care research must consider multiple causes and effects and identify the process whereby certain combinations of variables lead to certain outcomes. (p. 42)

Clinical reality is multidimensional. Multiple factors exist in a health care situation and affect the outcomes of care in different ways: independently, in combination, or interactively, thus forming a complex network of causes and effects. The multiple factors are related to the individual providing the care, to the person receiving the care, to the nature of the care given, and to the setting or conditions under which the care is given. Ignoring the contribution of these factors to the achievement of outcomes results in an inadequate understanding of what really goes on in the health care situation and how the outcomes are achieved. Furthermore, holding constant factors other than the intervention that might influence the outcomes expected of an intervention is neither possible nor informative under the natural conditions of clinical practice. The researcher's ability to control for the multiple factors is very limited; clinicians, rather than researcher, are in charge of the situation and may resist any change in practice, procedures, policies, or environment required for conducting the research study. Even if the researchers manage to control some of these factors, their study findings provide a simplistic and distorted representation of the intervention effectiveness, since in natural settings the effects of the intervention on the outcomes depend on these controlled factors. In addition, such findings may not be reproduced in another setting in which a similar experimental control is not feasible. Therefore, field researchers have to identify, incorporate, and empirically examine the effects of multiple factors on outcomes achievement. The theory-driven approach to effectiveness research is a strategy for achieving the goals of developing clinically relevant knowledge and building and testing practice-oriented theories.

THE THEORY-DRIVEN APPROACH
TO EFFECTIVENESS RESEARCH

In the previous two chapters, the limitations of the conventional, outcomes-focused approach to intervention effectiveness research were discussed. These limitations are related to the simplistic, black box approach to evaluating interventions, which focuses on determining whether the treatment works or does not work. The main concern is to demonstrate the causal connection between the intervention or program and the intended outcomes (Cook, 1993). The true experimental design is ideal for estimating the net effects of the intervention. Through random assignment, control of contextual factors, and manipulation of the treatment, extraneous factors that could influence the expected outcomes are controlled for. Controlling for these extraneous factors weakens the plausibility of alternative explanations of the observed treatment effects and enhances the validity of the causal connection.

The focus on the causal connection between the intervention or program and the outcomes detracts from validating the causal explanation of the intervention or program effects, that is, from determining why, how, and under what conditions the intervention is effective (Chen & Rossi, 1983; Cook, 1993). This simple causal connection ignores what goes on in the black box—that is, the complex causal processes mediating the intervention effects—making it difficult to interpret the findings. The assumption of "all things being equal" ignores (a) individual differences in the response to treatment, (b) variability in the amount of treatment received, (c) contextual variability, and (d) the humanistic aspect of treatment delivery. This assumption neglects the fact that even after randomization extraneous variables may still correlate with the intervention outcomes and that in a field or natural setting various factors interfere with the proper implementation of the intervention and therefore with the achievement of the desired outcomes (Chen, 1990; Chen & Rossi, 1983; Lipsey, 1990).

Shifting the focus of effectiveness research from causal connection to causal explanation is essential if the goal is to build the knowledge base for clinical practice and enhancing the quality of the care. Knowledge of the what, when, where, for whom, why, and how of a particular intervention facilitates its judicious utilization in or adaptation to varying clinical circumstances. Causal explanation requires theory. The theory models what goes on in a particular situation. It delineates the elements involved and the relationships among them. This chapter presents the theory-driven approach to intervention evaluation by focusing on the role of theory in effectiveness research. First, the types of theories needed for explaining the causal processes underlying an intervention effects are identified. Second, the elements and sources of theories are described. Third, the advantages of the theory-driven approach to intervention evaluation are presented. Points of discussion are illustrated with examples from the SHIP study.

Theory in Effectiveness Research

A theory is a broad attempt to organize and explain phenomena occurring in the world. The term *theory* "connotes a body of knowledge that organizes, categorizes, describes, predicts, explains, and otherwise aids in understanding and controlling a topic. Theories do this in many ways, such as searching for invariant laws, using definitions and axioms to deduce testable propositions, and describing the causal processes that mediate a relationship" (Shadish, Cook, & Leviton, 1991, p. 30). This conceptualization implies that a theory is a consistent group of statements that present a systematic view about phenomena occurring in real-life situations (Walker & Avant, 1989). The statements identify, define, and describe the phenomena involved in the situation, as well as specify the nature of the relationships among the phenomena. The purpose of theories is to describe and explain how and why some phenomena or events occur. Theories are ultimately used to organize and direct thought, observations, and actions. Intervention evaluation is concerned with understanding the why and the how of intervention effects. Therefore, theory in intervention evaluation has to explain the processes that mediate or condition the causal relationship between the intervention and the outcomes and specify the nature of the intervention and the procedures to be performed to bring about the desired effects (Chen & Rossi, 1989; Finney & Moos, 1989). Middle-range, descriptive theories are needed to describe two aspects of the clinical situation being assessed. The first aspect relates to the presenting problem for which treatment is given. The theory defines and describes the presenting problem (Lipsey, 1993) and models the processes that produce the presenting problem. The second aspect relates to the intervention. The middle-range theory identifies and describes (a) the causal processes through which the intervention is expected to produce the desired outcomes; (b) the expected effects of the intervention, that is, the specific changes expected as a result of the intervention; and (c) the conditions under which the causal processes will arise, that is, the individual, contextual, or environmental factors under which they occur (Chen, 1990; Lipsey, 1993). Practice, prescriptive theories are needed to specify what must be done to achieve the desired intervention effects. They provide information about the conceptualization and design of the intervention in terms of its purposes, components, intensity, and duration required to produce the desired outcomes; the human and material resources needed for delivering the intervention; and the procedures to be followed when implementing the intervention (Chen, 1990).

A specific intervention theory combines descriptive, middle-range theories and prescriptive, practice theories. Intervention theory is an attempt to explain why, how, and under which conditions the treatment effects occur. It consists of a set of statements regarding the nature of the intervention, the nature of the effects expected of the intervention, the processes mediating the expected effects, and the conditions affecting the intervention processes. Thus, an intervention theory is explanatory, providing for a clear understanding of what goes on when the intervention is implemented and which conditions facilitate or inhibit the effectiveness of the intervention; it is also action oriented, providing guidance on how to design and implement the intervention. An intervention theory need not be elaborate and detailed to be useful. Rather, it should be relevant in its content to the intervention being evaluated and it should be sufficiently explicit that its implications for intervention design, for research design, and for interpretation of findings can be carefully considered (Finney & Moos, 1989; Lipsey, 1993).

Elements of Intervention Theory

For an intervention theory to be useful in guiding the design of the intervention and of the evaluation study, it has to address the following elements: the problem for which the intervention is given, the critical inputs, the mediating processes, the expected outcomes, the extraneous factors, and implementation issues.

Problem Definition

"A problem definition . . . specifies which condition is treatable, for which populations, and under what circumstances, that is, a statement of boundaries that distinguish relevant from irrelevant situations" for the particular intervention or program in question (Lipsey, 1993, p. 11). Interventions address some problem representing actual alterations in functioning or inadequacies in the level of functioning with the potential of resulting in dysfunction. The presenting problem varies in its nature (i.e., actual vs. potential problem), manifestation, causative factors, and level of severity, among different client populations and under different conditions. Variations in the presenting problem require interventions with different purposes and consequently expected outcomes, rationale, structure, and strength or require modification or adaptation of an intervention with known efficacy. For example, dyspnea associated with anxiety requires an intervention that aims at reducing anxiety and consequently dyspnea; listening to sedative music may be appropriate in this situation. But dyspnea associated with excessive physical exercise requires an intervention to enhance breathing pattern and maximize oxygen availability; deep breathing or pursed-lip breathing may be more appropriate in this situation. Similarly, the same intervention may be appropriate and effective for different presenting problems. For instance, listening to sedative music is appropriate to relieve anxiety, pain, and agitation. In each of these cases, an intervention theory should describe the nature of the specific presenting problem for which the intervention is applied in terms of its manifestation, causative factors, and level of severity. The theory should also specify the client population experiencing the problem and identify the conditions under which the problem occurs.

An example from the SHIP study illustrates the elements of an intervention theory. The uncertainty in illness (Mishel, 1988) middle-range theory proposes that uncertainty is a problem experienced by persons with any illness and, if not managed properly, may interfere with the person's adjustment and adaptation. *Nature of the problem:* Uncertainty refers to a cognitive state of lack of form or structure to the events occurring in a specific illness condition. It is defined as the inability to determine the meaning of illness-related events. *Client population:* Although uncertainty is experienced by diverse client populations, uncertainty as experienced by women with breast cancer is of interest here. *Conditions:* In women with breast cancer, uncertainty is experienced at different phases of the cancer experience or in relation to different events, such as diagnostic procedures, surgical treatment, adjuvant therapy, and side effects of cancer therapy. Of particular interest in the SHIP study is the uncertainty experienced in association with adjuvant therapy, which is often given intermittently over a specified period of time. *Manifestations:* Women with breast cancer experience multiple side effects of cancer and its therapy, such as fatigue, sleep disturbance, and pain. These symptoms are aversive, discomforting, distressful, and unfamiliar; they may be incongruent or inconsistent with the women's expectations. Therefore, the women may not be able to interpret them or understand their meaning and their impact, resulting in uncertainty. Uncertainty is a cognitive state than can take four forms: (a) ambiguity concerning the state of illness, (b) complexity regarding treatment of care, (c) lack of information about the diagnosis and seriousness of the illness, and (d) unpredictability of the course of the disease and prognosis. Uncertainty is perceived as being either a danger or an opportunity—that is, uncertain events that lack clarity and predictability are viewed as difficult to manage and therefore dangerous or harmful. Coping methods, directed at reducing uncertainty, are used. When the uncertainty of events is appraised as more beneficial than a definite negative state, the uncertainty becomes a preferable state and coping methods to maintain uncertainty are used (Mishel). *Causative factors:* Uncertainty results when illness-related events are perceived as lacking familiarity, specificity, consistency, or completeness. It is "created when the person cannot adequately structure or categorize an event because of the lack of sufficient clues" (Mishel, 1988, p. 225). In particular, uncertainty is generated by (a) the occurrence of symptoms in an inconsistent manner that makes it difficult to recognize a pattern attributable to the disease or its treatment; (b) the novelty or lack of familiarity of events in the health care environment, such as the initiation of a new treatment; (c) the lack of congruence between what is expected and what is experienced, such as the treatment failing to produce the expected outcomes by a predetermined time; (d) lack of knowledge about the disease, its treatment, and its impact and about adjustment and coping strategies; (e) altered information-processing abilities associated with the disease or its treatment that influence the individual's interpretation of events; (f) lack of social support or interaction with others (discussion and supportive interactions with others provide an opportunity to clarify the situation, to interpret events, and to share strategies for handling various threatening events); and (g) lack of trust and confidence in the health care providers (Mishel, 1988). In women with breast cancer, uncertainty is related to any of the following concerns: (a) specific concerns about cancer diagnosis, such as the stage of cancer, metastasis, and recurrence; (b) concerns related to cancer treatment efficacy and outcomes; (c) concerns related to responses to side effects of treatment; (d) concerns related to living with cancer, such as family's responses and concerns and self-image; (e) concerns related to caring for self, such as ability to function in desired or expected roles and ability to cope with the illness- or treatment-related changes; and (f) concerns about daily life, such as employment, financial issues, and changing lifestyle. *Level of severity:* The severity of uncertainty is determined by the extent to which the concerns are appraised as threatening or dangerous or as an opportunity.

Specification of Critical Inputs

The critical inputs address the nature of the intervention in terms of what is necessary to produce the expected effects. The critical inputs delineate the practical, prescriptive aspect of the intervention theory in terms of what should be done (Chen, 1990; Lipsey, 1993). They define the components constituting the intervention, the mode of delivery, and the strength or dosage of the intervention required to bring about the desired changes. The critical inputs guide the implementation of the intervention; they specify the activities to be performed for delivering the intervention, and they detail the procedures to be followed and the amount, frequency, and duration of the intervention activities. The uncertainty management intervention (UMI) in the SHIP study was developed by Mishel, based on the uncertainty in illness theory. Mishel designed the UMI to reduce uncertainty by addressing its causative factors and its manifestations. The intervention consists of four phases: problem identification, appraisal of the uncertainty, appraisal of the meaning of uncertainty, and delivery of interventions to manage the uncertainty (McHenry, Allen, Mishel, & Braden, 1993). The *problem identification phase* focuses on identifying the specific concern(s) about which the woman feels uncertain (i.e., specific concerns or concerns related to treatment, to response to treatment, to living with cancer, to caring for self, and about daily life, as presented earlier). The *appraisal of uncertainty phase* is concerned with defining and specifying the particular aspect of the concern that is associated with uncertainty, as well as how the uncertainty is manifested. The particular aspect of the concern could be the illness-related event experienced by the women (such as the specific symptom), its meaning, its outcome and consequence, and its management. For instance, the women may express concerns related to the experience of fatigue (Does it result from the illness or its treatment? Does it mean that I am getting worse?), to the outcome of fatigue (How is it going to affect me?), and to the management of fatigue (I do not know what to do about this fatigue). Uncertainty is then manifested by the women perceiving the concern as conflictual, inconsistent, unpredictable, unfamiliar, having multiple meanings, and lacking structure or by the women lacking adequate knowledge or information about it. The *appraisal of the meaning of uncertainty phase* focuses on identifying what the uncertainty means to the client: Is it appraised as danger or opportunity for growth? The appraisal is divided into levels of low, moderate, and high danger, as well as opportunity, with corresponding criteria defined for each level. Once the problem area, causes, and manifestations of uncertainty are identified, the fourth phase of the UMI consists of *delivering interventions to manage uncertainty*. The interventions for managing uncertainty have cognitive, psychological or emotional, and behavioral components. The cognitive component is composed of interventions designed to (a) strengthen an existing cognitive structure and reinforce appraisals of uncertainty as an opportunity for growth (e.g., reinforcing the women's coping strategies and validating their self-care behaviors), (b) promote cognitive structure formation such as providing information to the women and assisting in anticipatory planning and problem solving, and (c) reduce negative certainty when negative certainty is inappropriate or incorrect (e.g., promoting an opportunistic view of the situation). The psychological component includes interventions that regulate the emotional response of the women by encouraging positive self-talk, ventilation of feelings, and selective use of humor. The behavioral component aims at managing continual uncertainty by enhancing personal control and encouraging probabilistic thinking. An assessment/appraisal/ intervention protocol that describes the steps constituting each phase of the UMI and provides a list of concerns and interventions is available to guide the delivery of the intervention. The protocol also specifies the mode for delivering the UMI. Since the causative factors and the manifestations of uncertainty are individualistic, varying across clients, the UMI is to be delivered individually and interactively, through a telephone contact. During the phone contact, a semistructured interview format is used to explore the women's concerns and appraisal of uncertainty and to deliver the intervention(s). The intervener and client engage in an open, unhurried discussion of emerging concerns, in which the intervener inquires about the women's status through investigative, open-ended questions; evaluates the women's perceptions of the situation; identifies the uncertainty-related problem expressed by the women through reflective comments and clarification of the content of the message with the women; and provides the most appropriate intervention, selected from the protocol list, to manage the particular problem identified. The concern(s) identified for each woman and the intervention(s) delivered are recorded on a computerized form of the assessment/appraisal/intervention protocol. The computerized form permits easy access to the information and serves as a basis for reassessment, determination of resolved problems, identification and appraisal of new areas of uncertainties, and selection of new interventions at subsequent phone calls. The dosage of the UMI is defined by the total number of phone contacts made over the 6-week period following the initiation of adjuvant therapy. The women are expected to experience uncertainty during this period due to the novelty of the events occurring, such as the initiation of treatment, the experience of new symptoms, and the contact with the health care providers and the health care system (which may be unfamiliar to some women). Therefore, they require assistance in managing their uncertainty. The interveners are expected to make a total of six phone calls for each woman over a period of 6 weeks, with an average of one phone call per week. The women are also invited to call the intervener during the week to discuss emerging problems. The length of the phone call is not limited to a predetermined number of minutes; rather, it is a function of the number of concerns identified, the number and nature of the intervention(s) delivered, and the ability and willingness of the women to disclose her concerns (McHenry et al., 1993).

Mediating Processes

Mediating processes refer to the "links, phases, or parameters of the transformation process that the treatment brings about, the intervening or mediating variables on which the process is contingent" (Lipsey, 1993, p. 11). The processes represent the series of changes that occur in the participants after the delivery of the intervention and that yield to the expected outcomes. The series of changes can be depicted in the form of a causal model or in a stage-state model.

A causal model represents the hypothesized relations among key mediating variables reflecting the causal processes underlying the intervention effects. A causal model is used when the changes reflect alterations in the level of some attributes that are sequentially linked to the desired outcomes. The causal chain Intervention → Knowledge → Behavior illustrates a causal model depicting the mediating processes of an educational intervention. The mediating processes underlying the effects of the UMI can be depicted in a causal model. Based on the intervention theory, it is hypothesized that (a) the UMI cognitive component increases the women's knowledge related to the disease and its treatment and strengthens their cognitive structure or cognitive reframing skills, which promote their appraisal of uncertainty as a challenge for growth rather than as danger; (b) the UMI psychological component reduces their emotional distress associated with the illness and its treatment; and (c) the UMI behavioral component enhances their ability to manage uncertainty. The ultimate outcomes of the UMI are reduced uncertainty and improved psychological adjustment. Figure 3.1 summarizes the processes mediating the effects of the UMI (Braden et al., 1989; Mishel, 1990).

A stage-state model represents the major stages through which the persons progress toward achieving the desired status. This kind of model is used when the changes reflect transitions through discrete stages culminating in the achievement of the desired outcome. The chain Intervention

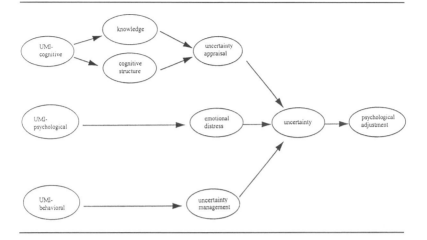

Figure 3.1: Processes Mediating the Effects of the UMI

→ Stage 1 → Stage 2 → Ultimate Outcome state illustrates a stage-state model underlying an intervention effects (Lipsey & Pollard, 1989). The transtheoretical model of change is an example of a stage-state model. The transtheoretical model proposes that cessation of high-risk or addictive behaviors and the acquisition of health-promoting behaviors involve the progression through five stages of intentional change: (a) precontemplation: persons have no intention to change behavior, (b) contemplation: persons are seriously thinking about the change but have not yet made a commitment to take action, (c) preparation: persons are intending to take action in the next month, (d) action: persons are in the process of changing their behavior and are committed to it, and (e) maintenance: persons continue to work on the change in behavior to prevent relapse (Prochaska, DiClemente, & Norcross, 1992).

Specification of Expected Outcomes

The expected outcomes include the various intervention effects. They represent the changes in the clients' health status resulting from the intervention. The intervention theory specifies the nature of the anticipated outcomes, the expected timing at which the changes are expected to occur, and the expected pattern of change in the outcomes after the delivery of the intervention, as well as any hypothesized interrelationships among the outcomes (Chen, 1990; Lipsey, 1993). *Nature of outcomes* refers to the particular aspect of the clients' health status that the intervention impacts, such as self-care abilities and physical, mental, or social functioning. The nature of outcomes is determined by the presenting problem and the purpose and mediating processes underlying the intervention. The timing refers to the point in time at which the changes occur after implementing the intervention. Some changes occur immediately after the intervention delivery, whereas others take some time to appear (Lipsey, 1993). The immediate outcomes could represent the changes mediating the impact of the intervention on the desired, ultimate outcomes.

For example, increased knowledge is expected to occur soon after the implementation of the UMI, as illustrated in Figure 3.1, since the intervener gives the women information about their illness, treatment, or side effects of cancer therapy during the phone contacts. The knowledge provided by the intervener is learned and is therefore expected to be maintained over time. Thus, the change in knowledge following the UMI takes on a nonlinear pattern, characterized by an abrupt increase in the level of knowledge gained that remains at the same level at subsequent points in time, as illustrated in Figure 3.2 (Sidani, 1994). With increased knowledge, the women put the event causing the uncertainty in context and provide meaning to it; they then perceive it as less threatening, thereby reducing uncertainty. Changes in the management of uncertainty require some time to appear since the women are exposed to the management strategies during the phone contacts and need opportunities to apply them before they can use them successfully. Therefore, significant changes in this outcome may not be detected immediately following the delivery of the UMI.

Extraneous Factors

Extraneous factors include contextual or environmental factors and client characteristics that significantly affect treatment processes and consequently the intervention effectiveness in achieving the desired outcomes (Lipsey, 1993, p. 11). These factors may operate in two ways: (a) they may influence the outcomes directly; and (b) they may moderate the intervention effects where the effects of the intervention on the outcomes are conditional on the level of the extraneous factors—that is, the effects of the intervention on an outcome differ under different conditions or vary as the

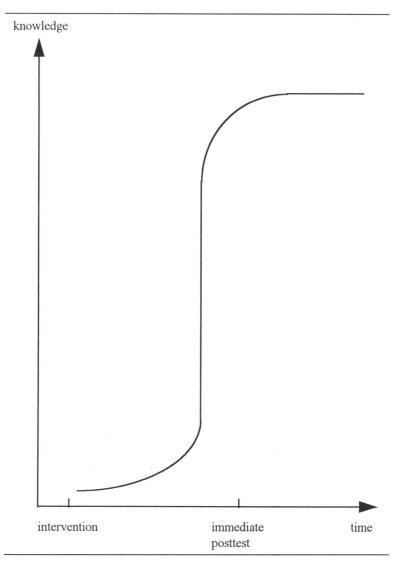

Figure 3.2: Pattern of Change in Knowledge Following the UMI

extraneous factor takes on different values (Chen & Rossi, 1987; Costner, 1989; Finney & Moos, 1989).

Based on the uncertainty in illness theory and on empirical findings, education and anxiety are factors that affect the effectiveness of the UMI.

Education is proposed to have a direct influence on uncertainty, which is an intended outcome. Individuals with a lower level of education report higher levels of uncertainty, are able to modify the uncertainty less rapidly, and experience uncertainty for longer periods of time than individuals with more education (Christman et al., 1988; Mishel & Braden, 1988). Education also influences the response pattern to the UMI since individuals with less education require more time to construct meanings for events (Mishel, 1988) and demonstrate least knowledge gain following educational programs (Gierszewski, 1983). Anxiety is also moderately but positively associated with uncertainty (Wong & Bramwell, 1992). Furthermore, it can moderate the UMI effect on knowledge. Anxiety influences knowledge gain by altering the individuals' cognitive capacity: It results in attentional deficits that block cognitive processes needed for learning (Duryee, 1992; Meisenhelder, 1987; Mishel, 1988).

Implementation Issues

Implementation issues include "aspects of the treatment delivery system relevant to its function of providing the specified treatment" (Lipsey, 1993, p. 11). They refer to the resources required for carrying out the intervention activities. The resources relate to the setting, equipment, and personal and professional characteristics of the intervener that facilitate the delivery of the intervention as originally designed. For instance, the resources needed for implementing the UMI were phone, computer, computerized protocol form, and private room to maintain privacy during the phone conversation. In addition, the interveners selected to provide the UMI needed (a) to have experience in the areas of oncology and psychosocial nursing in order for them to conduct a comprehensive assessment and identify the women's concerns, and (b) to demonstrate attentive listening and effective communication skills (McHenry et al., 1993).

All elements of an intervention theory must be identified and described when evaluating the effectiveness of a particular intervention. In general, the greater the specificity in the conceptualization of the intervention, the easier the design and the delivery of the intervention will be, the better the ability to maintain the integrity of its implementation, and the greater the ability to identify and isolate factors that could confound or obscure the intervention effects. As a result, the specificity of the effects is increased, which improves the validity of conclusions (Trochim, 1985).

Sources of Theory

Intervention theory can be obtained from various sources, based on the extent of knowledge available within the topical area. The development of an intervention theory can be either deductive, when the intervention theory is derived from prior substantive theory or from prior effectiveness research findings, or inductive, when the intervention theory is built by exploring the framework underlying the intervention being evaluated.

Health professionals base their understanding of the clinical problems and consequently the interventions to address them on available substantive theories, on their clinical experience, or on the results of previous studies examining the clinical situation or the effectiveness of similar interventions. A substantive theory attempts to explain the clinical situation: It describes the presenting problem, it identifies the factors causing the problem and explains the linkages among these factors and the presenting problem, and it points to the consequences of the presenting problem. A clear understanding of the problem directs professionals to possible treatments for resolving it or preventing its consequences. Such an understanding of the problem determines the mechanisms through which the treatment is expected to resolve the problem; that is, it determines the changes in the key mediating variables that should be induced by the treatment to resolve the problem (Rossi & Freeman, 1993). Thus, the explanation of what the treatment is and how it should work forms the basis for deriving the treatment theory. When well-developed substantive theories are not available, professionals resort to findings of previous studies examining the problem or the intervention of concern. From these findings, a conceptual framework presenting a tentative explanation of the processes underlying the treatment effects and specifying the nature of the intervention can be developed.

When a well-defined theoretical or conceptual framework cannot be identified, such as when professionals are dealing with a relatively new clinical situation or with a situation that has not been well studied empirically, they resort to their initial understanding of the situation or problem gained through their clinical experience. The professionals develop interventions from their initial understanding of the problem and working hypotheses of how the treatment is expected to work. The rationale underlying these interventions is usually implicit and probably not clear or well established. Making the rationale explicit is necessary for an informed evaluation of the intervention effectiveness. Qualitative and exploratory research methods could be used "to attempt to bring to the surface those concepts and linkages that are implicitly assumed" by the clinicians involved in designing or delivering the intervention of interest (Lipsey & Pollard, 1989). Qualitative methods consist of reviewing the intervention protocol and conducting in-depth interviews with those involved in planning and implementing the intervention. The interviews are geared toward obtaining the clinicians' understanding and perception of how the intervention is supposed to work, of the nature of the intervention, of what the expected outcomes are, and of the ideal conditions for the intervention to be effective. Clinical examples documenting the success of the intervention can be sought during the interviews. The data obtained are content-analyzed to define the key operating variables, such as extraneous, process, and outcome variables, and to identify the relationships among these variables. The emerging framework can be developed into an intervention theory, grounded in the data (Strauss & Corbin, 1994). Alternatively, exploratory studies can be conducted to collect preliminary, rather descriptive, data on an intervention. Case studies and observational inquiry are useful in assessing the design of interventions and programs; in describing their methods of delivery, the role of the intervener, and the participants' responses; and in identifying factors that might influence the treatment effects. Results of these exploratory studies can be organized into a framework that attempts to describe the processes underlying the intervention effects and to specify the critical inputs of the intervention (Lipsey & Pollard, 1989).

Advantages of Intervention Theory

The advantages of identifying and explicitly stating the intervention theory in effectiveness research are numerous. An intervention theory guides the development, design, and delivery of an intervention and the design of an effectiveness study, improves the validity of findings, and enhances the clinical applicability of the intervention.

Design and Delivery of the Intervention

A well-defined intervention theory guides the design and delivery of the intervention. With a clear understanding of the presenting problem and consequently of the reasons for using the treatment and of the processes underlying its effects, professionals are able to identify the critical inputs of the intervention. Specification of the critical inputs (i.e., components, activities, strength) and description of the implementation issues facilitate the development of the intervention protocol and the delivery of the intervention as planned. A priori knowledge of how the treatment should be delivered helps the researcher in planning process evaluation and monitoring the integrity of intervention implementation. Monitoring treatment delivery assists in identifying sources of implementation problems and highlighting variability in the treatment components and strength or dosage that can be tolerated (i.e., what treatment dose, precise estimate or range of levels, is still effective in achieving the intended outcomes? Do differences in the dosage of the treatment received result in the intended effects? What is an acceptable range of these differences?). Being aware of implementation problems is necessary for a valid interpretation of findings, for developing strategies to cope with these problems, and for improving future application of the treatment in various field settings. Thus, the integrity of treatment implementation is enhanced, and the chances for Type III error (i.e., concluding that an intervention is not effective when it has not been implemented as designed) are reduced (Hoefer, 1994; Sechrest, Ametrano, & Ametrano, 1983; Yeaton, 1985). Learning about the acceptable range of dosage is important for determining the extent to which modifying the intervention to meet the individual needs of clients will produce the desired effects (Chen & Rossi, 1989; Lipsey, 1990).

Design of Effectiveness Study

An intervention theory guides the design of an effectiveness study. Theory is the basis for informed choices about research methods (Lipsey & Pollard, 1989). A theory helps in

1. Identifying the target population and selecting the sample of participants. Participants who do not have the presenting problem for which

the intervention is given obviously cannot be helped by the treatment being evaluated, no matter how effective.

2. Identifying participants' subgroups for whom the intervention may have differential effects.

> Some treatments affect everyone about the same; others are apt to have varying effects depending on the circumstances and characteristics of each recipient. In the latter cases, there is a variety of subpopulations for whom the treatment-outcome relationships may differ. Failure to distinguish among them misrepresents the treatment effects and muddies an understanding of the nature of treatment benefits. To find such patterns of differential response, measures must be included for those subject characteristics likely to interact with the treatment. (Lipsey, 1993, p. 17)

> The intervention theory informs about which subjects' characteristics have the potential of moderating the intervention effects. These characteristics are then specified as criteria for inclusion or exclusion. If included, meaningful characteristic × intervention interaction terms are created and empirically tested.

3. Identifying the study variables and appropriate measures. An intervention theory specifies the intervention and key mediating and outcome variables in the particular situation of interest. The theory also provides for a careful definition of these variables that makes possible an appropriate operationalization of these variables and therefore enhances construct validity (Chen & Rossi, 1987; Trochim, 1985).

4. Specifying the appropriate time(s) for measuring the outcome variables. The intervention theory predicts which effects occur at what point in time and proposes the pattern of change in the outcomes over time, thus dictating the points in time at which the outcomes should be measured and the period of time required for a meaningful follow-up (Lipsey, 1993).

5. Delineating the relationships among the treatment, mediating, and outcome variables, which dictates the proper statistical model for data analysis and produces efficiency in data analysis. That is, the theory tells what analyses to do or relationships to test, thus reducing Type I error associated with repeated statistical testing (Cohen, 1982; Sechrest, 1986). Furthermore, the theory points to the expected size of the intervention effects, which helps in examining the clinical significance of findings.

Validity of Conclusions

Intervention theory plays a major role in dealing with the various types of validity of an intervention evaluation study. Contrary to the conventional approaches to enhance validity, each focusing on one type of validity only, intervention theory has the advantage of addressing internal, statistical conclusions, construct, and external validity simultaneously and of improving the study sensitivity in detecting real intervention effects. The theory prespecifies the factors with the potential to threaten the internal validity of a study. Extraneous factors related to the characteristics of participants, interveners, and setting; having a direct effect on the intervention outcomes; or correlated with the treatment variables (i.e., components and dosage) are identified. Assuming that their potential influence on the outcomes is neutralized or held constant through randomization or experimental control may be inappropriate. Extraneous factors continue to vary after randomization (Chen & Rossi, 1987; Cook & Campbell, 1979; Costner, 1989). Therefore, once identified in the intervention theory, they can be measured and later modeled in the statistical analyses. Testing for the extraneous factors' effects on the intervention and its outcomes is a useful strategy for examining the plausibility of alternative hypotheses explaining the study findings, rather than simply guessing what could have influenced the effectiveness of the intervention. That is, testing for these effects provides empirical evidence for ruling in or out threats to internal validity. The influence of extraneous factors on outcomes, whether direct or through a correlation with the treatment, is manifested by a differential subject response to the intervention, thereby introducing variability in the outcomes that could not be accounted for by the treatment; thus, it contributes to error variance in tests of statistical significance. By including the relevant extraneous factors in the model explaining the intervention effects, a certain percentage of the variance in the outcomes is attributed to these factors, thereby reducing error variance. With reduced error variance, real intervention effects are more likely to be detected (Lipsey, 1990).

The intervention theory enhances the validity of statistical conclusions. The theory predicts the expected effect size, which assists in determining the sample size required for an effectiveness study. The theory specifies the relationships to be tested; it guides statistical analyses and reduces the problem of "fishing in the data" and the associated Type I error (i.e., concluding that the intervention is effective when in fact it is not). Thus, there is greater confidence that findings that corroborate the hypotheses are not due to chance alone. Furthermore, including the extraneous factors in the analysis reduces error variance and minimizes Type II error (concluding that the intervention is not effective when in fact it is, but its effects were obscured by the influence of extraneous factors) (Chen & Rossi, 1987; Cohen, 1982). Finally, intervention theory defines the intervention carefully and prespecifies the relationships between the treatment variables (including the mediating variables and the intervention components and strength). Empirically testing for these relationships requires monitoring the integrity of the intervention implementation and measuring the intervention-related variables and including them in later analyses. Measuring the intervention variables involves collecting data on the type and dosage of the intervention received by participants in the experimental and control groups. This strategy permits assessment of the extent of "slippage" and of diffusion and imitation of the treatment, which, in turn, reduces the likelihood of Type I and III error and rules in or out one threat to internal validity, that is, diffusion of treatment.

Intervention theory improves construct validity of a study. A theory clearly and specifically defines the variables of interest, which enhances the operationalization of constructs. Thus, the construct validity of measures is maintained. Measures that are construct valid are more sensitive to the "real" intervention effects (Lipsey, 1990). Furthermore, intervention theory prespecifies how factors related to the subjects, setting, interveners, and intervention are interrelated and how they influence the achievement of intended outcomes. Examining these relationships assists in determining and controlling for, at least statistically, confounding constructs, thus enhancing the validity of findings (Chen & Rossi, 1987).

Intervention theory identifies which of the extraneous factors moderates or conditions the effectiveness of the intervention in producing the expected outcomes. These moderating effects mean that "an observed effect under one condition does not occur (or does not occur to the same degree or in the same direction) under some alternative condition" (Costner, 1989, p. 347). Therefore, examining interaction effects of extraneous factors with the treatment variables (such as subject × intervention and setting × intervention) determines the client population for whom or the conditions under which the intervention is or is not effective, thereby improving generalizability or external validity of the findings (Chen & Rossi, 1987).

An intervention theory distinguishes between the theoretical framework and the delivery system of an intervention. The distinction between the theoretical and methodological framework of the intervention facilitates the interpretation of findings. When the findings indicate nonsignificant effects, intervention theory guides the investigators in their search for "what went wrong." Failure to demonstrate significant effects can be related to failure of the research design, failure or inadequacy of implementation, or failure of the intervention theory. The role of intervention theory is to provide a framework that permits judgment of the plausibility of these alternative explanations of the nonsignificant findings. When the findings support the effectiveness of the intervention in achieving the intended outcomes, intervention theory provides for a clear understanding of what exactly produced the effects and on which parameters of the situation the results are contingent. It explains how the intervention works and establishes limits on the generalizability of the effects (Lipsey, 1993).

Clinical Applicability

Intervention theory provides for a causal explanation of the observed intervention effects. With an adequate understanding of the processes linking the intervention to the outcomes and of the factors that condition, facilitate, or hinder these processes, it becomes much easier to generalize the results to other populations, treatments, and settings (Conrad & Conrad, 1994; Judd & Kenny, 1981). Inadequate knowledge and explanation of the causal processes underlying the achievement of desired patient outcomes "leads to what Weick calls 'superstitious learning' in which, because a consequence follows an action, one assumes that the action lead to the consequence, when, in fact, there is no causal connection between them all" (Mark, 1995, p. 45). Knowledge of the how and why enhances the clinical applicability of the research findings: "Such knowledge permits treatment to be applied in an intelligent and responsive fashion rather than in a mechanical or stereotyped form. . . . When only the empirical fact is known, the treatment can only be reproduced as a ritual in the hope that it will have the expected effects" (Lipsey, 1993, p. 10). In other words, the results of a theory-driven effectiveness study provides knowledge of which specific component of the intervention, with which dosage, under what conditions, results in which outcomes, for which client population. Such knowledge consolidates the theoretical basis of clinical practice that is used by clinicians to prescribe the most appropriate care for clients, thus improving the quality of the care provided.

Operationalizing the Theory-Driven Approach

The advantages of theory in effectiveness research make the theory-driven approach to intervention evaluation appealing to investigators and clinicians. The theory-driven approach to effectiveness research consists of developing an intervention theory that provides causal explanations of the intervention effects, of developing a framework for evaluating the intervention effectiveness that is derived from the theory, and of designing and conducting the study accordingly (i.e., as guided by the theory and the framework).

The framework is suggested as a strategy for operationalizing the intervention theory. The framework represents the elements of the intervention theory as variables and proposes relationships among them. The framework incorporates variables related to the intervention, to the processes mediating the intervention effects, to the outcomes expected of the intervention, and to extraneous factors influencing the intervention effects. The intervention variables include the component(s) of the intervention and its dosage as actually received by the participants. The mediating variables are those linking the intervention variables to the outcomes expected of the intervention. The extraneous variables include client, intervener, and setting-related characteristics that may influence the effects of the intervention.

The framework is based on three assumptions. First, it is assumed that individuals' self-select their entry into treatment and into the type and dosage of treatment received. The individuals' characteristics influence self-selection, which, in turn, leads to differential response to treatment. Second, it is assumed that the intervention does not necessarily have equal effects on all individuals receiving it. The response to the intervention varies between individuals. Third, variability in the responses to the intervention can be explained in light of multiple causes, including the intervention and extraneous factors.

The major propositions of the framework are the following:

1. The clients' characteristics influence the manifestation and level of the presenting problem, which, in turn, influences the type and dosage of the treatment to be given.
2. The client, setting, and intervener-related variables influence the outcomes expected of an intervention in different ways: (a) direct relationships with the outcome variables; (b) indirect effects, whereby they affect the type and dosage of the treatment received by participants and subsequently the response to treatment; and (c) conditioning effects; whereby they weaken or potentiate the intervention effects.
3. The intervention variables influence the mediating variables.
4. The mediating variables influence the intermediate outcomes and subsequently the ultimate outcomes.

This framework is comprehensive and complex. It depicts the complexity of real life, in which multiple factors affect the achievement of the outcomes expected of an intervention or program. It incorporates multiple variables, both theoretical and practical, that contribute to the intervention effects, as specified in the integrative descriptive and prescriptive intervention theory. Taking these factors into consideration and empirically testing for their impact enhances the validity of effectiveness study findings, reflects the complexity of clinical reality in which networks of multiple causes and multiple effects operate, and increases the understanding of the processes underlying the intervention, all of which promote its applicability in clinical practice. The elements of this framework are discussed in detail in the following chapters.

Chapter 4

CHARACTERISTICS OF CLIENTS

Health-related interventions and programs are designed and delivered to relieve a presenting problem, prevent it from occurring, or promote a desirable state (Eisenhauer, 1994). A systematic, empirical evaluation of intervention effectiveness requires that the intervention be given to individuals who are experiencing the specified problem treatable by the intervention or at risk of developing the untoward condition. Therefore, the problem to be treated or avoided forms the most important criterion for selecting potential participants in an intervention effectiveness study. In the conventional experimental approach to effectiveness research with a focus on outcomes, additional criteria for sample selection are imposed in an attempt to control for some extraneous factors that may influence the intervention effects. These additional criteria pertain to the characteristics of individuals with potential influence on the expected outcomes. This chapter focuses on the factors related to the client that influence the outcomes of interventions. The role of client characteristics is analyzed. The types of client characteristics and the nature of their influence on outcomes are described. Conventional strategies for dealing with client characteristics are examined, and their limitations in developing clinically relevant knowledge are discussed. Finally, alternative methods for empirically determining the influence of client characteristics are presented and illustrated with examples taken from the literature and from the SHIP study. The advantages and disadvantages of these methods are discussed.

The Role of Client Characteristics

Human beings differ from each other on various qualities or characteristics. These interindividual differences reflect the unique constitution of the person in terms of physiological and physical functioning, affect, behavior, attitude, beliefs, values, cognitive processes, cultural norms, and psychosocial functioning. Individual differences in these characteristics affect the clients' general susceptibility to illness; the nature and extent of the presenting problem; the design and selection of interventions; the clients' beliefs, values, and preferences for treatments; and the clients' response to illness and to treatment.

There is growing evidence that social and environmental conditions influence the clients' overall health and susceptibility to illness. For example, social support was found to decrease mortality from various causes, risk for depressive symptoms, incidence of heart disease in men, and cancer incidence and mortality in women (Heller, 1990). There is also accumulating evidence that the individuals' definition of health, value for health, beliefs about health and illness, biologic and demographic characteristics, and perceived self-competence affect their level of engagement in health-promoting lifestyles; lifestyles, in turn and in combination with situational factors, determine the health status experienced at a certain point in time (Frank-Stromborg, Pender, Walker, & Sechrist, 1990; Johnson, Ratner, Bottroff, & Hayduk, 1993). Any actual or potential alteration in health status is the presenting problem that clinicians attempt to resolve or prevent through interventions. Individual differences in client characteristics yield variability in the nature and extent of the presenting problem. Therefore, clients entering treatment are unique, varying on different characteristics.

Individual variability in the nature and extent of the presenting problem determine the design of the intervention or the selection of the intervention to be delivered. The influence of client characteristics on the design and selection of the intervention can be illustrated by the prescription of different types or doses of antibiotics to treat an infection in different age groups; by having the clients choose a music selection, based on their individual preference, to induce relaxation; by the need to adapt a diet regiment to the cultural preferences of the client; and by the need to alter the content, activities, or teaching methods and mode of delivering an educational intervention to fit the clients' learning style.

The effects of beliefs, values, and preferences for treatments are widely acknowledged by clinicians, but these effects have not been studied systematically until recently. Results of studies indicated that clients who dropped out of care were younger; of lower socioeconomic status; of low educational level; had low knowledge of the disease, its consequences, and the benefits of the prescribed treatment; and had minimal support from family members or significant others (Caldwell, Cobb, Dawling, & de-Jough, 1970; Deyo & Inui, 1980; Finnerty, Mattie, & Finnerty, 1973). Warnecke et al. (1991) conducted a study to describe factors associated with participation in televised smoking cessation programs. Three types of interventions were made available to potential participants: televised program segments broadcast in the evening, manuals sent by mail or distributed at some centers, and support group meetings that participants attended with a self-selected nonsmoker buddy. The smoking cessation programs were advertised on television during the evening news. Interested viewers were requested to contact the nearby research center for more information about the programs. Over 325,000 smokers were exposed to the program at some level. The design was quasi-experimental, with participants self-selecting their treatment of choice. A random sample of residents in the area in which the programs were implemented were interviewed by phone. The results of logistic regression analyses indicated that the characteristics of those who participated in the various interventions differed as follows: (a) those who viewed the televised segments tended to be females (odds ratio = 1.29) of low income (odds ratio = 1.57); (b) those who used the manual tended to be heavy smokers (odds ratio = 1.02); and (c) those who attended the support group meetings tended to be nonblack (odds ratio = 1.15), older (odds ratio = 1.64), and of high income (odds ratio = .24 for low- vs. high-income groups).

The influence of individual characteristics on the clients' response to illness or to treatment is becoming of increasing interest to researchers. For instance, Mumford, Schleisinger, and Glass (1982) found that (a) postsurgical mortality rate was highest among clients who were slightly depressed prior to surgery; (b) a high level of preoperative fear was associated with slower recovery, greater use of analgesics, and more negative emotions after the surgery; and (c) hopeful and cooperative patients tend to have a smoother and swifter recovery from illness than depressed and uncooperative patients.

In conclusion, interindividual differences in various aspects of life and health are normative. These differences result in variability in the way people respond to treatment and therefore in their ability to achieve the desired outcomes of care.

Types of Client Characteristics

In intervention effectiveness research, client characteristics are of concern because of their potential influence on the response to treatment. Although numerous client characteristics could influence achievement of desired outcomes, those of particular interest when evaluating health-related interventions or programs are categorized into personal characteristics, illness- or health-related characteristics, and resources available to clients.

Personal characteristics include variables related to demographics, to personality traits, to emotional status, to cognitive processes, and to personal and health beliefs and values. Examples of personal characteristics are age, gender, education, ethnicity, anxiety, resourcefulness, sense of mastery, learning style preference, and depression. Illness- or health-related characteristics consist of variables that indicate the severity of illness, such as staging of illness, perceived symptom burden, functional status or ability to perform activities of daily living, and the number of symptoms experienced (Brooten & Naylor, 1995; Jones, 1993). Resources available to clients consist of internal and external factors that provide clients with the support needed to carry out the intervention as prescribed. Examples of resources are variables such as availability of social support, employment, health care cost coverage, income, and coping strategies. This list of client characteristics is preliminary rather than comprehensive or exhaustive. Furthermore, the classification of client characteristics presented here (i.e., personal, health, resources) is not prescriptive or definitive; there are multiple ways of categorizing a particular client characteristic. For instance, health beliefs can be categorized as personal characteristics or as resources available to clients. The identification and categorization of client characteristics with a potential influence on the response to treatment are based on the intervention theory, findings of the initial or pilot test of the efficacy of the intervention, findings of studies evaluating interventions with similar components, and clinical observations.

Effects of Client Characteristics in Effectiveness Research

Diverse client characteristics can influence health in different ways, two of which are of particular relevance when evaluating interventions. First, client characteristics may influence the nature, course, and manifestation of the presenting problem and therefore the selection and design of interventions. Second, client characteristics can influence the clients' response to the intervention.

Individual client characteristics may lead to variations in the nature and underlying etiology of the presenting problem and in its manifestation. The presenting problem may be associated with different causative factors in different client populations. For example, Hawkes and Holm (1993) found that men and women differed in cardiovascular risk factors (men were more likely to have smoked or to have a history of heart disease whereas women were more likely to be obese) and in factors that prompt them to engage in physical exercises (women held more favorable attitudes toward exercise whereas social influence from doctors, health experts, and spouses was a strong predictor of exercise participation in men). Rossi and Freeman (1993) presented the example of homelessness to illustrate the importance of defining and understanding the presenting problem when designing and evaluating social programs. They proposed that homelessness could be explained by two different underlying mechanisms. One mechanism identifies the homeless persons as those who have no relatives or significant others on whom to be dependent; the other mechanism defines homelessness as the lack of access to shelter. "The first definition centers attention primarily on the social isolation of potential clients; the second focuses on housing arrangements" (Rossi & Freeman, 1993, p. 61). Lack of kin or social support system and lack of resources are individual characteristics responsible for the presenting problem in this example. Examples illustrating the influence of client characteristics on the manifestations of a presenting problem are abundant in the clinical literature. For instance, the level of state anxiety is a function of age, with younger persons experiencing more anxiety than their elders (Lundeman, Asplund, & Norbeg, 1990; Payne, 1992).

A clear definition of the presenting problem and identification of its underlying causative mechanisms provide direction to the clinicians or researchers designing or choosing the intervention that is most appropriate for remedying the problem in a particular client population (Adelman, 1986). Appropriate interventions are those that target the underlying etiology or manifestation of the problem as identified in the target population (Eisenhauer, 1994). The results of Hawkes and Holm's (1993) study examining exercise participation in men and women have some implications for designing exercise-promoting interventions. For instance, social influence should be part of exercise-promoting interventions for men and not for women. The intervention could be designed to target the spouses or health care providers of male participants. The intervention could consist of encouraging the spouses of male participants to participate in the exercise program and to provide continuous support, and of asking the health care providers to procure reinforcement to male participants to improve their adherence to the exercise program (Hawkes & Holm, 1993). In Rossi and Freeman's (1993) homelessness example, the design of social programs directly follows the explanations given for the homelessness situation: "The first definition might lead to a program that attempts to reconcile homeless persons with their alienated relatives; the second, to a subsidized housing program. Thus, the two problem definitions lead to quite different proposed programs" (Rossi & Freeman, 1993, pp. 61-62). More studies examining the effectiveness of specific interventions for specific patients are needed.

Client characteristics can influence the achievement of the outcomes expected of the intervention or program. Client characteristics influence outcomes directly and indirectly. The direct effects are represented by a direct path between the client characteristic and the expected intervention outcome (see Figure 4.1, Part A). The direct effect of the client characteristic, which is considered an extraneous variable, on the intervention outcomes indicate that the interindividual variability in the outcomes observed at posttest is a function of the client characteristic. Therefore, this direct effect would lead to either (a) a smaller effect size than theoretically expected, since a proportion of the variance in the posttest outcome has been accounted for by the client characteristic; or (b) a significant effect size as theoretically expected, but the observed effect is attributable to the client characteristic rather than to the intervention. Consequently, the validity of conclusions regarding the effectiveness of an intervention is

A. Direct Effect

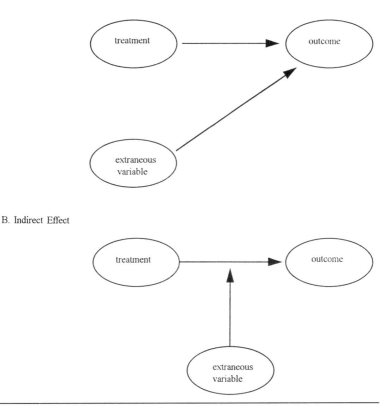

B. Indirect Effect

Figure 4.1: Influence of Client Characteristics on Outcomes Achievement

threatened (Costner, 1989). For instance, the age of participants should be taken into consideration when evaluating the impact of a psychoeducational intervention on life satisfaction, since a positive correlation between age and life satisfaction has been reported (Campbell, 1981). Thus, variability in life satisfaction observed at posttest can be explained, at least partially, by age rather than the intervention. Similarly, variability in physical functioning observed after the delivery of an intervention designed to enhance self-care abilities and skills can be explained by initial (i.e., pretest) or concurrent level of severity of illness.

The indirect effects of client characteristics on the intervention outcomes can take the form of an interactive or conditioning effect between a
particular client characteristic variable and the intervention variable (see
Figure 4.1, Part B). The interactive effect indicates that the effect of the
intervention on the outcomes differs under different conditions of the
characteristic (Finney & Moos, 1989). It is reflective of differential responses to treatment observed in different subgroups of the participants;
the subgroups are differentiated on the basis of their level on a characteristic
of interest. The interactive effect takes three forms. First, the interaction
effect is observed under one condition (such as high level of the client
characteristic) and not under some alternative condition (such as low level
of the client characteristic). Second, the effect does not occur to the same
degree under the different conditions, such as observing a moderate effect
when the level of the characteristic is high and a very low effect when the
level of the characteristic is low. Third, the effect does not occur in the same
direction under different conditions, such as finding an increase in the
outcome level when the level of the characteristic is low and a decrease in
the outcome level when the level of the characteristic is high (Costner,
1989). In other words, an interactive effect implies that the client characteristic moderates the intervention effects, either potentiating or strengthening, or weakening or nullifying them. Integrative literature reviews and
meta-analyses have contributed significantly to the identification of differential treatment effects, as they permit systematic analysis of substantive
factors affecting the observed intervention effectiveness (Glass, McGaw,
& Smith, 1981). Brown (1992) found that patients' age influenced the strength
of the effects of educational interventions designed to improve knowledge,
self-care behaviors, metabolic control, and psychological status in adult
diabetic patients. The effect size estimates were considerably smaller for
groups primarily over the age of 40 years. Gallagher-Thompson and Steffen
(1994) conducted a study to examine the differential effects of cognitive-
behavioral and brief psychodynamic interventions on depression in caregivers of elders. A significant treatment × length of caregiving interaction
effect was noted, indicating that short-term caregivers (< 44 months) improved more in the brief psychodynamic condition and longer term caregivers (> 44 months) improved more in the cognitive behavioral condition.
    Significant client characteristic × intervention interactive effects have
some implications for the external validity and clinical applicability of the
effectiveness study findings. Significant interactive effects imply that the

intervention is not equally effective in all subgroups of the target client population; rather, the intervention produces the desired effects in a particular group of clients who have a specific level of the conditioning or moderating characteristic. Therefore, the generalizability of the study findings to the full range of target clients is limited. Similarly, the intervention cannot be automatically prescribed to any member of the target population without assessing his or her standing on the conditioning characteristic. Knowledge of which client characteristic moderates the effects of the intervention leads to judicious prescription and delivery of the intervention in real life, whereby the most appropriate intervention is given to clients who would most benefit from it. Such practice enhances the efficiency and quality of health care services.

In summary, there is some clinical and preliminary empirical evidence suggesting that client characteristics play major roles in a health care situation. They contribute to the definition of the presenting problem, to the choice of intervention, and to the response to the intervention. In effectiveness research, client characteristics are often viewed as extraneous factors threatening the validity of the causal connection between the treatment and the outcomes since they create initial group nonequivalence that obscures the treatment effects. Therefore, researchers must be aware of strategies for dealing with client characteristics properly to enhance the validity of conclusions. These strategies are classified into two broad categories: the conventional strategies that attempt to eliminate their effects and alternative strategies that attempt to determine their effects.

Conventional Strategies for Dealing With Client Characteristics

Client Characteristics as Threats

In the conventional method for evaluating the effectiveness of an intervention, the primary concern is to validate the causal connection between the intervention delivered and the intended outcomes, as described in the earlier chapters. Factors other than the intervention that might affect the subjects' response to the intervention are considered threats to the validity of the intervention-outcomes causal relation.

Individual client characteristics can result in initial differences between study participants. Initial differences in the outcomes occur either between the experimental and the control groups or within the experimental group. Between-group differences are likely to be associated with nonrandom assignment of subjects to the experimental and control groups. They present as variability in the level of outcomes at pretest, whereby one group has a higher or lower mean score on the outcome measure than the other. Thus, the initial between-group differences are systematic, resulting in bias. They may have a direct impact on the outcomes, causing significant differences in the posttest outcomes between the groups. Client characteristics causing between-group differences *obscure* or *mask* the effects of the intervention. They weaken the confidence in attributing postintervention differences between the groups to the intervention, since posttest differences are associated with the initial differences on the outcome variable or with the client characteristic that created the initial differences rather than the treatment. The statistical analysis in effectiveness research aims at determining if the treatment produced the expected outcomes. Usually, an analysis of variance is performed to determine if group membership (i.e., receiving versus not receiving the intervention) makes a difference in the outcome(s), above and beyond what would have been expected by chance alone. Within this context, chance reflects the naturally occurring individual differences on the outcomes. The analysis of variance F-ratio tests for differences between the experimental and control groups by comparing between-group variance to within-group variance. Between-group variance represents the differences in the outcome variable between the experimental and control groups. Within-group variance represents the individual differences in the outcome variable. Therefore, any differences in the groups' mean values on the outcome variable that are associated with pretest differences in the groups or with client characteristics increases the between-group variance. This large difference between the means of the experimental and control groups leads to biased findings: It results in overestimation of the treatment effects and misinterpretation of the findings since the observed differences are incorrectly attributed to the treatment at a time when they should be attributed to the client characteristic.

Client characteristics may lead to initial within-experimental group differences in the outcomes variable despite random assignment and careful selection. The within-experimental group individual differences influence the participants' response to treatment, which is manifested by variability in the level of the outcomes achieved posttest. This variability in outcomes reflects personal differences in the response to treatment that cannot be explained by group membership. Therefore, increased within-group variance reduces the value of the F-ratio (Lipsey, 1990), indicating that group membership does not make any difference in the outcome, above and beyond the individual differences. This implies that participants in the experimental group are unique in their response to the outcomes measure or responded differently, in their own idiosyncratic way, to the intervention.

Client characteristics can moderate intervention or program effectiveness in producing the desired outcomes, manifested by differential treatment effect in subgroups of clients with different levels on a characteristic. This differential intervention effect translates into a significant intervention × characteristic interaction term, which threatens the external validity of the study findings.

In summary, client characteristics result in individual differences in the outcomes variables. These differences can lead to (a) large between-group differences that are not causally linked to the intervention and therefore induce bias in estimating the intervention effects, and (b) increased individual variability in the outcome that weakens the statistical power to detect significant intervention effects and that limit the generalizability of the findings. Consequently, client characteristics present alternative explanations of the study findings, whether the findings are significant or not.

Strategies for Controlling Client Characteristics

Within the experimental framework, client characteristics leading to differences on the outcomes must be controlled for to eliminate their influence. This control aims at making individuals assigned to the experimental and control groups as equivalent as possible prior to the application of the intervention (hereafter called initial equivalence), so that any posttest differences in the outcomes between the groups can be confidently attributed to the causal effect of the intervention (Rubin, 1974). Initial group equivalence refers to similarity of the groups' mean pretest values on any characteristic that creates differences in the groups in the absence of a treatment effect and on any characteristic that may affect the posttest scores. Thus, initial group equivalence is an indispensable criterion for validity within the experimental framework (Reichardt, 1979). Methods for controlling client characteristics are categorized into experimental and statistical control methods.

Experimental Control

The primary purpose of the experimental control methods is to ensure initial group equivalence. Controlling for clients' characteristics is executed in two ways: careful sample selection and random assignment to groups (Cook & Campbell, 1979; Keppel, 1991). The sample selection criteria serve two functions: excluding clients with characteristics having the potential to confound the intervention effects and reducing the subject heterogeneity or variability on the outcomes. Selecting clients into an effectiveness study is based on a set of well-defined inclusion and exclusion criteria. In an intervention evaluation study, participants are sampled primarily on the basis of experiencing the problem amenable to treatment by the intervention and possessing the characteristics representative of the target population with the potential of benefiting from the intervention. The exclusion criteria are of utmost importance, as they represent the client characteristics that may create interindividual differences within and between the experimental groups that could mask or potentiate the intervention effects. For instance, in the SHIP study, the inclusion criteria included women with breast cancer; 18 years of age or older; able to read and write English; and currently receiving adjuvant therapy for breast cancer on an outpatient basis, including chemotherapy, radiation therapy, hormone therapy, or hyperthermia, independently or in combination. These inclusion criteria cover the characteristics of the target population with the presenting problem that the SHIP interventions are designed to resolve. Women with breast cancer receiving adjuvant therapy experience physical and emotional distress, potentially leading to problems in psychological adjustment. The self-help interventions were designed to assist these women in managing their needs and daily care and in improving their psychosocial adjustment and well-being. Women with clinically diagnosed psychopathology, such as major depression, were excluded from the study, because psychological alterations interfere with learning, with perception of events, and with performance of self-care activities, which were considered the major outcomes of the self-help interventions.

Random assignment of selected participants to the experimental and control groups is intended to increase the likelihood that participants in the two groups are similar and that the influence of potential extraneous factors, such as client characteristics, is dispersed across the groups.

Random assignment is used to make the groups equal on all measured and unmeasured variables, thus reducing selection bias or systematic between-group differences not accounted for by the intervention:

> Assigning units to conditions on a chance basis means that units with a given idiosyncracy which are assigned to one group will, on the average, be counterbalanced by units with comparable (but not necessarily identical) idiosyncrasies in the other group. . . . Randomization does not, of course, remove idiosyncracy from any one unit. . . . But prior to the treatment and after random assignment, the average score of all the persons in a particular group should not differ from the average score in the other group. Hence, the pre-test means of the different treatment groups should not differ. (Cook & Campbell, 1979, p. 344)

Statistical Control

There are instances in which random assignment is not possible due to ethical issues or is not carried out correctly. There are also instances in which careful sample selection and random assignment are not successful in ensuring initial group equivalence. In fact,

> The equivalence achieved by random assignment is probabilistic. Thus it is not inevitable that a correctly implemented randomization procedure will result in groups that do not differ. Obviously, with a small initial sample of persons who differ widely on a dependent variable of interest, random assignment may result in dissimilar groups. . . . Even with large samples and dependent variables of low variability, the pre-test means will not be identical, and statistically significant differences will sometimes be obtained by chance alone. (Cook & Campbell, 1979, pp. 341-342)

In simpler terms, sample selection and random assignment do not guarantee initial group equivalence and do not guarantee lack of interference of individual differences on the posttest scores. Random assignment

> does not 'control' for the extraneous variables by holding them constant. They continue to vary and hence continue to have their effects on 'outcomes,' thus adding to the error variance (i.e., the variance in 'outcome' not associated with 'treatment'). This may have serious consequences in that a higher error variance reduces the power of any test of statistical significance of the relation between 'treatment and outcome.' Otherwise

stated, with higher error variance we are in greater danger of failing to recognize an effect when it is there. (Costner, 1989, p. 346)

In situations in which the groups are not initially equivalent or when a client attribute is believed to influence the posttest scores, experimental researchers resort to methods allowing for a statistical control of these nuisances. The analysis of covariance (ANCOVA) permits examination of between-experimental group differences after removal of additional sources of variation in the outcomes variable. The additional sources of variation in the outcomes could be related to either initial differences in the outcomes (i.e., pretest scores) or extraneous factors (i.e., client characteristics correlated with the outcomes). ANCOVA addresses the question of whether the experimental group outperformed the control group on the posttest by more than should be expected on the basis of initial differences or of differences related to extraneous client characteristics (Munro & Page, 1993; Reichardt, 1979) by adjusting the posttest scores for these initial individual differences. Thus, ANCOVA is used to improve the equivalence of the experimental and control groups prior to determining the effectiveness of the intervention. ANCOVA partials out individual differences observed initially or associated with client characteristic(s); it does not permit examination of how and to what extent the client characteristic(s) affect outcomes achievement, however. The latter case requires other strategies, discussed in subsequent sections.

ANCOVA tests for treatment effects in a two-step procedure:

Step 1. The client characteristic that influences the posttest outcome is identified. Its identification is theoretically or empirically based. Theoretically, the client characteristic that influences the intervention effectiveness is derived from the intervention theory or framework guiding the effectiveness study, as described in Chapter 3. In the absence of a well-defined intervention theory, the client characteristic is identified empirically either from findings of previous effectiveness studies or from finding significant differences in the mean pretest outcome scores between the experimental and control groups or finding nonsignificant differences in the mean posttest outcome scores between the two groups. Thus, the characteristic, called covariate, could be the pretest score on the outcome or any client characteristic. The covariate must have been measured during the study and must be correlated with the outcome, based on theoretical prediction or previous empirical findings. Once the covariate is identified, its effect on the posttest outcome of interest is estimated by regressing the posttest outcome values on the covariate scores.

The regression analysis estimates the regression parameters in the total sample. The obtained numerical values of these parameters are then used to estimate a value of Y, the outcome, for each subject, called the predicted-Y. The predicted-Y represents the posttest outcome score based on the subject's level on the covariate, regardless of the subject's group membership. Next, the deviation of the subject's actual score on the outcome from his or her predicted outcome score is calculated. These deviations are then used to compute the error term of the F-ratio. These deviations are expected to be smaller than those obtained in a traditional one-way analysis of variance (ANOVA) since the individual variability in the posttest outcomes related to the covariate has been accounted for.

Step 2. The means of the experimental groups are also adjusted for group differences on the covariate. The adjustment consists of calculating the mean for each experimental group based on its mean covariate value. The adjusted means and error term are then used in an ANOVA F-ratio to determine the effect of the treatment (Keppel, 1991).

The advantage of the ANCOVA technique is that it increases the study sensitivity in detecting significant intervention effects. In the traditional analysis of variance, the total variance in the dependent variable is partitioned into between-group variance, representing the treatment effect, and error variance, representing variability that is not accounted for by the treatment. Therefore, any additional variability associated with extraneous factors, such as client characteristics, is lumped into the error variance component. With increased error variance (i.e., the denominator of the F-ratio), the F-ratio value is decreased, indicating no significant intervention effects. In an ANCOVA model, the total variance in the dependent variable is partitioned into between-group variance, variance associated with the covariate (note that more than one covariate can be used), and error variance (Wildt & Ahtola, 1978). By allowing for individual differences due to the covariate of concern and residualizing the variance attributed to the client characteristic from the total variance, the error variance is reduced. With reduced error variance, the chances of detecting group differences are increased.

Despite its advantage in reducing error variance and improving the study sensitivity to detect intervention effects, if present, ANCOVA does not examine how the extraneous factors, that is, the client characteristics, influence the clients' response to the intervention. ANCOVA permits estimation of the strength of the relationship between a single covariate or a set of covariates and the posttest outcome measure, but, in clinical situations, more than one client characteristic may be operating at the same time, each having a differential effect on the outcomes. Furthermore, the effect of the covariate(s) may be different in the various experimental groups being compared, a reality that is inconsistent with the ANCOVA assumption that the relationship between the covariate and the dependent variable is similar in each group. Also, ANCOVA estimates the direct relation between the covariate and the outcome measured at posttest, but its model falls short of examining any interactive effect of the covariate $\times$ treatment on the outcomes, as the covariates are assumed not to be correlated with the independent variable and their effects are residualized in the first stage of the ANCOVA procedure (Keppel, 1991). Knowing which factor or client characteristic(s) modifies the effects of an intervention on which outcomes is essential for learning about who would benefit most from the intervention. Such knowledge provides the basis for clinical decision making (Crano & Messe, 1985).

It may be argued that determining which client characteristic modifies the response to treatment is a step undertaken after demonstrating that the intervention is efficacious—that is, the investigators have first to show that the intervention produced the desired outcomes, indicated by significant differences in the outcomes between the experimental and control groups, under relatively controlled conditions (i.e., controlling for extraneous factors). Then, they move to the next step of examining which client characteristic influences outcome achievement in subsequent effectiveness studies (i.e., in the real world) and how. Although this sequence of studies is ideal, it may not be always possible, especially when the results of the first efficacy study indicate that the intervention is not effective. The point we emphasize here is that extraneous factors, such as client characteristics, may have moderated or weakened the intervention effects and that the conclusions about the intervention effects, drawn from the first efficacy study, may be invalid. Therefore, the influence of client characteristics should be recognized as a potential threat to the validity of the inferences in an efficacy study, even though the random assignment procedure was carefully followed; the influence of client characteristics should be systematically examined, as these characteristics are considered substantive factors of clinical relevance.

Alternative Strategies for Dealing With Client Characteristics

Client Characteristics as Substantive Factors

There is growing need, expressed by researchers and clinicians, to progress from evaluating the effectiveness of interventions in producing the desired outcomes under controlled conditions to conducting such evaluation studies in real-world settings in an attempt to develop clinically relevant knowledge and enhance the generalizability of findings to clinical practice (Erben, Franzkowiak, & Wenzel, 1992). Clinical knowledge informs clinicians who would benefit most from the intervention.

The development of clinically relevant knowledge demands some changes in the conceptualization of and methodology for studying the effectiveness of interventions. First, the complexity of the clinical reality must be acknowledged and examined. The simplistic, reductionistic representation of the causal connection between an intervention and its effects needs to be expanded to reflect the complex network of causes and effects. The model guiding an effectiveness study has to incorporate all substantive factors influencing the expected intervention outcomes (Chen & Rossi, 1987; Costner, 1989). The substantive factors presented in this chapter are the client characteristics: demographic, personal, health or illness related, and resources available. Second, the uniformity assumptions (initial equivalence on characteristics and equal response to treatment) of the traditional experimental framework are not congruent with clinical reality. Clients are unique in their characteristics and their response to the intervention. Therefore, it cannot be assumed that they enter treatment with the same characteristics or that the intervention will have a uniform impact across clients. Rather, interindividual differences due to client characteristics must be acknowledged and modeled and empirically examined (Caplan, 1968; Daro & McCurdy, 1994; Marfo & Dinero, 1993; Shonkoff et al., 1988). Client characteristics influence intervention outcomes in two ways: They can have direct effects on the expected intervention outcomes or they can moderate the intervention effects.

Strategies for Examining the Effects of Client Characteristics

The methods available for determining the effects of client character-istics on intervention outcomes are analytical or statistical, involving modifications of the set of study variables and the relationships examined rather than experimental modifications in the study design. Thus, they can be used whether the design is true or quasi-experimental. In true experi-mental studies, examining the influence of client characteristics is advo-cated when (a) the randomization procedure was not successful in equal-izing the groups or was not followed faithfully, resulting in initial group nonequivalence; (b) the researcher knows, a priori, that a specific client characteristic affects the clients' response to treatment; or (c) the findings indicate a statistically nonsignificant difference between the experimental groups in which individual differences related to some attributes are primarily responsible for the findings.

When the client characteristic is identified a priori, the researcher may elect to use a *randomized block design*. In this design, subjects are first separated into groups, or blocks, according to their scores on the specified blocking variable, which could be either their pretest scores on the outcome measure or their standing on the characteristic. Then, subjects in each block are randomly assigned to the experimental and control groups (Jacobson & Christensen, 1996; Reichardt, 1979). In quasi-experimental field studies, examining the influence of client characteristics is important for enhancing the validity of conclusions since they were not controlled for through randomization. By measuring the extraneous variables and incorporating them into the analysis, the power of statistical tests to detect significant effects is increased (Chen & Rossi, 1987; Costner, 1989). Two alternative methods are discussed next: blocking and individual regression analysis.

Blocking

Blocking in quasi-experimental field studies differs from the blocking used in randomized block designs. It is done a posteriori during data analysis rather than when assigning participants to groups. The purpose of blocking is to control for initial interindividual differences. Blocking consists of dividing the subjects into subgroups representing different levels of the attribute responsible for initial differences in the outcomes. It involves three steps. The first step consists of identifying the variable on the basis of which the subgroups are formed. The variable is derived from the intervention theory or from empirical findings. This variable is called the blocking variable and includes any characteristic responsible for the individual differences between the subjects, such as the pretest score on the outcome measure or other attributes (personal, health related, and resources). In the second step, the subjects are divided into subgroups on the basis of their score on the blocking variable. Subjects in both the experimental and the control group are ranked and placed into subgroups that have similar scores on the blocking variable. Thus, the subjects within the subgroups are homogenous relative to their level on the blocking variable (e.g., high vs. low level). In the third step, the blocking and the treatment group membership variables are entered in the statistical analyses as independent variables affecting the outcome. A two-way analysis of variance is performed to test the effects of the treatment, the effects of the blocking variable, and the effects of the interaction term treatment × blocking variable on the posttest outcome measured at either one point in time or repeatedly over time.

In an intervention evaluation study, the outcome variables are measured at least once before and after the treatment implementation. In some situations, the outcomes are measured before and on several occasions after treatment implementation. For instance, when a control group could not be included for comparison, researchers resort to repeated measurement of the outcomes posttest to increase the reliability of findings. In such situations, the pattern and amount of change in the outcomes over time are of interest. Client characteristics may influence the pattern or amount of change in outcomes. In the blocking method, the influence of the blocking variable on the pattern or amount of change in outcomes can be determined by using a mixed-design analysis of variance. This complex analysis of variance incorporates between-subject and within-subject factors. The between-subject factors include the treatment variable and the blocking variable; the within-subject factors include time. The time factor represents the changes in the outcome scores over the occasions of measurement. The interaction effect of blocking variable × time can be tested. A significant block × time effect implies that the average pattern of change in the outcomes differs across the blocking subgroups (e.g., in one subgroup the mean outcome score increases over time whereas in another it decreases).

The advantages of the blocking method include, first, decreased subject heterogeneity on the posttest outcome measure. In this analysis, the total variance in the outcome measure is partitioned into the variance accounted for by the intervention, the variance accounted for by the blocking variable, and the error variance. Thus, the variance attributed to the blocking variable is subtracted from the error variance, resulting in reduced error variance (Reichardt, 1979). As a result, the statistical power to detect significant intervention effects is increased. A second advantage is estimation of differential intervention effects on posttest outcomes within each level of the blocking variable, detected with the interaction of the blocking × treatment term. Exploring differential treatment effects enhances external validity of findings through identifying subgroups in the population for whom the treatment is or is not effective. In addition, examining differential treatment effects answers the clinical question of which client population would benefit most from the intervention evaluated.

Researchers considering using blocking as a strategy for determining the effects of client characteristics on intervention outcomes need to be aware of two issues. First, the blocking variable can be either categorical, such as gender, or continuous, such as age. When the blocking variable is categorical, the analysis becomes very similar to the factorial, or two-way, analysis of variance, in which the blocking variable and the group membership variable are the two factors. But when the blocking variable is continuous, the researchers have to create the blocking subgroups based on some cutoff score, such as the median of the blocking variable. The practice of dichotomizing a continuous variable

> throws away information because individuals within a subgroup are treated as if they were identical with respect to the attribute in question, when there is evidence to the contrary. This loss of information typically reduces measurement precision, underestimates the magnitude of bivariate relationships, and lowers statistical power for detecting true effects. . . . [Further] dichotomizing continuous predictor measures may in fact lead to overestimates of strength of relationship accompanied by an increase in Type I errors, that is, to results that are spuriously statistically significant. (Maxwell & Delaney, 1993, p. 181)

Second, the number of blocking variables that can be used in any analysis is very limited (usually one blocking variable is used at a time), thus restricting the ability to represent the set of client characteristics that may influence the intervention outcomes simultaneously in actual clinical situations. Conducting repeated analyses to examine the effect of several blocking variables increases the chances of committing Type I error. Despite its advantage in determining differential response to the intervention based on a characteristic of interest, the blocking method is still conducted at the subgroup level, since the subjects are divided into smaller groups, and differences between these groups are examined with an analysis of variance. In the analysis of variance, the individual idiosyncratic responses are considered a source of error. But it is exactly these individual responses that are of interest to clinicians. Therefore, what is needed is a method to examine the influence of client characteristics on the pattern of change in the outcomes, at the individual level.

Individual Regression Analysis

Individual regression analysis (IRA) was originally developed to examine the individual patterns of change on some attribute over time (Burchinal & Appelbaum, 1991). The pattern of change is described by a trajectory or curve that reflects the rate at which the individual's value on the attribute changes over time (Francis, Fletcher, Stuebing, Davidson, & Thompson, 1991). The IRA framework adopts an idiographic perspective in which uniqueness in the trajectory of change are acknowledged. Thus, the primary purpose of IRA is to investigate individual differences in change by describing the intraindividual pattern of change and inquiring about potential characteristics predicting interindividual differences in the pattern of change (Nesselroade, 1991). IRA addresses the question, What kind of person changes at what rate? Examining the pattern of change in the individuals' level on outcome over time is a means for evaluating the effectiveness of the intervention. The application of IRA in effectiveness research requires that (a) longitudinal data are available in which the outcome variable has been measured on more than two occasions on all individuals, and (b) the outcome variable retains the same meaning over the occasions of measurement. If different things are measured at each point in time, using different instruments or the same instrument, then it becomes difficult to infer change since the question becomes, Change in what? (Burchinal & Appelbaum, 1991; Rogosa, Brandt, & Zimowski, 1982).

In effectiveness research, IRA is particularly helpful in investigating systematic interindividual differences in the pattern of change in the outcomes, that is, differences in the pattern of change related to individual client characteristics can be explored. IRA involves two steps.

Step 1. The pattern of change is described for each individual subject. The pattern of change refers to the rate at which the subject's value on the outcome variable changes over time. It is represented by a curve or line that reflects the functional relationship between the values on the outcome variable and time. This functional relationship can be delineated by a regression equation, in which the subject's value on the outcome is regressed on the time variable:

$$Y_{it} = B_0 i + B_{1i} X_{it} + R_{it},$$

where Y_{it} is the predicted subject's value on the outcome variable measured over time; $B_0 i$ is the intercept and describes the value on the outcome variable at baseline (or when the time variable is zero); B_{1i} is the slope and describes the direction and rate of change in the outcome variable, for each individual, over time; X_{it} is the time variable representing the occasions of measurement (incremental numerical values are assigned to the different occasions of measurement); and R_{it}, is random error in the outcome variable, for each individual, at a specific point in time; it includes both error of measurement and error of prediction (Rogosa & Willett, 1985). The slope is the most important parameter to be evaluated in an intervention effectiveness study as it indicates the rate of change in the outcome over time. The slopes are evaluated for direction and magnitude. Negative slopes imply that the values on the outcome decrease with time; positive slopes imply that the values increase with time. Slopes with values greater than .70 indicate that the values on the outcome variable change rapidly; moderate slopes (between .30 and .60) indicate that the values on the outcome change slowly over time; slopes with values less than .30 indicate no significant change.

In IRA, the functional relationship between outcome and time described in this individual regression equation is linear, represented by a straight line. A straight line indicates a constant rate of change, meaning that the value on the outcome changes by a certain amount (defined by the slope) at each point of measurement. Nonconstant rate of change, represented by an S-shaped curve, for instance, can be represented by using the appropriate transformations, such as polynomials or logarithmic regression equations (Rogosa & Willett, 1985).

The same model of change (i.e., same regression equation) is applied when defining the pattern of change for each individual subject. The rate of change is individually estimated, however—that is, even though a linear pattern of change is assumed for all subjects, the actual rate of change may differ across the subjects. Different types of functional relationships can be used for individuals in the different experimental groups (Burchinal & Appelbaum, 1991; Rogosa & Willett, 1985).

IRA does not require the same data collection design for each individual. The number and spacing of measurement occasions may vary across persons, since the focus is on the true process of change (Bryk & Raudenbush, 1992; Francis et al., 1991). This makes IRA appealing in situations with data missing on different subjects on different occasions.

Step 2. Individual slopes are regressed on the intercept estimated in Step 1 (representing initial interindividual differences), the treatment, the client characteristics, and the interaction between them. As in multiple regression, the contribution of each predictor and the explanatory power of the regression model can be examined.

The principles underlying individual regression analysis are consistent with the clinical perspective that emphasizes the uniqueness of clients. The pattern of change in the outcomes is examined for each subject, thus providing detailed information of how each participant responds to the intervention. Furthermore, the direct and moderating effects of client characteristics on the response to treatment are estimated, which is informative in identifying clients that benefit most from the intervention.

In the SHIP study, the direct and moderating effects of selected client characteristics on the outcomes were investigated using individual regression analysis. The selected client characteristic was sense of mastery, defined as the belief in one's self as capable of influencing outcomes of one's own behavior and of overcoming life's adversities. In previous studies, a significant relationship was found between sense of mastery and knowledge acquisition, which is expected of psychoeducational interventions (Lowery & DuCette, 1976). It was hypothesized that sense of mastery would have a direct effect on cancer-related knowledge gain and would moderate the effect of the interventions on knowledge gain. Individual regression analysis was conducted to test these hypotheses. In the first step, the pattern of change in knowledge was described for each of the 56 participants who remained across the six points of data collection. The slopes for knowledge ranged between −.60 and 2.8, with a mean of .69 for the total sample, .88 for the combined intervention group, .64 for the uncertainty management group, .71 for the self-help classes, and .56 for the control group. In the second step, the direct and moderating effects of sense of mastery on knowledge were tested using multiple regression. Only the sense of mastery × experimental group membership interaction effect was statistically significant, accounting for 7% of the variance in knowledge gain. Based on the coding scheme used to represent the experimental group, this interaction effect indicates that women who received the combined intervention or the uncertainty management intervention and who had a high sense of mastery gained most in cancer-related knowledge, that is, a high sense of mastery strengthened the effects of these two psychoeducational interventions on knowledge but did not have any additional impact on the effects of the self-help classes (Sidani, 1994). Thus, these two interventions were most beneficial in improving knowledge of cancer and its treatment for women with high sense of mastery or control over events.

Summary

Throughout this chapter, the importance of examining the effects of client characteristics on the outcomes expected of an intervention was emphasized. The client characteristics may have direct effects on outcomes achievement whereby they mask the intervention effectiveness or indirect effects whereby they moderate its impact. The particular characteristic to be studied and the nature of its influence on outcomes are specified by the intervention theory. Examining the characteristic effects has statistical and substantive advantages. Determining the effects of client characteristics on intervention outcomes reduces error variance and increases the statistical power to detect significant intervention effects. Testing for their moderating effects permits examination of differential responses to treatment, thus improving the understanding of how and for whom the intervention works and the external validity of the findings. It also assists in building clinically relevant knowledge. The knowledge gained from this analysis addresses the clinical question, Who would benefit most from the intervention?

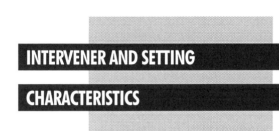

Chapter 5

INTERVENER AND SETTING CHARACTERISTICS

Clinical experience and preliminary empirical evidence suggest that the personal and professional attributes of clinicians affect the technical and interpersonal aspects of care. The technical aspect of care refers to the services provided by the clinician to produce the desired outcomes. The interpersonal aspect of care refers to the way clinicians relate to patients. The technical and interpersonal aspects of care have a direct impact on outcomes of care. Similarly, the physical and psychosocial characteristics of the setting in which the health care situation takes place influence the nature of and the method for delivering health services, which, in turn, affect outcomes of care (Donabedian, 1980; Tarlov et al., 1989).

In effectiveness research, the intervention is delivered by selected interveners in particular settings. Differences in the interveners and the settings result in variability in the way the intervention is implemented and in the way clients respond to the treatment, thus leading to increased variability in the outcomes achieved that is not attributed to the intervention effects. The characteristics of the intervener and of the setting have the potential of threatening the validity of conclusions regarding the intervention effectiveness. In this chapter, the effects of the intervener and setting characteristics on the intervention outcomes are discussed. Conventional and alternative strategies for handling them are presented.

Intervener Characteristics

The term *intervener* refers to the health care professionals—clinicians or researchers—involved in the delivery of the intervention being evaluated. Practitioners and researchers are individuals who differ from each other on various characteristics and thus cannot be assumed to be equal in who they are, what they know, what they do, and how they do things.

Types of Characteristics

Clinicians vary in their personal and professional characteristics. Personal characteristics include attributes related to demographics, personality traits, and interpersonal style. Examples of personal characteristics are age; gender; ethnicity; communication skills; demeanor, including friendliness, courtesy, sensitivity, being gentle and understanding, tone of voice, and body language; appearance, including attractiveness, neatness, and method of presentation; maturity; emotional well-being; perceptual and cognitive style; expectancies; and economic incentives. Professional characteristics include the skills needed for properly carrying out the activities making up the intervention. Examples of professional characteristics are educational background, discipline, and specialty training; level of competence or expertise in the clinical area pertinent to the intervention being implemented; beliefs and attitudes toward health and health care; preferences for treatment modalities; manual dexterity; and job satisfaction (Beutler, 1991; Bond & Thomas, 1992; Epstein, 1995; Tarlov et al., 1989). This list of personal and professional characteristics is by no means exhaustive.

Influence of Intervener Characteristics in Effectiveness Research

In studies evaluating the effectiveness of an intervention, the intervener is the medium through which the intervention is delivered to participants. The specific role and responsibilities, the extent of her or his involvement in implementing the treatment, and the degree to which she or he interacts with the participants during the treatment phase depend on the nature of the intervention. For instance, if the intervention consists of having the clients listen to music while sitting comfortably in a recliner, the intervener's role may be limited to providing clients with the music tape, the earphones, and the tape player; instructing them on how the equipment functions; and telling them to sit comfortably in the recliner and relax. The intervener may stay with the clients while listening to music or may leave the room. Thus, the intervener has minimal interaction with the participants. Providing health education is a more complex intervention in which the intervener assumes the following responsibilities: preparing a lesson plan, leading the discussion, and attending to the particular needs expressed by some participants while ensuring that the whole content is covered as planned in the time allotted for the session. Here, the intervener is involved in the different activities constituting the intervention and in a dynamic interaction with the participants during the sessions.

Interventions must be implemented as planned for their intended effects to take place. Providing the intervention as planned relies on the interveners' understanding of the essential features of the intervention and on their technical and interpersonal skills in carrying out its specific activities. For the interveners to implement the intervention properly and as faithfully as possible to the original design, they need to be aware of the presenting problem and its causative factors, the objectives of the intervention, its underlying theoretical framework, its expected outcomes, and the procedures to be performed in delivering it. This information must be given to the intervener, especially when the intervention is complex and is based on the individual clients' needs requiring some decision making on the part of the intervener. In addition to understanding the intervention, the interveners must possess the skills required for carrying out the specific activities constituting the intervention.

The particular skills and characteristics needed for delivering the intervention are dictated by the intervention theory. The intervention theory delineates the components of the intervention, its activities, its mode of delivery, and the resources needed to carry out the intervention activities. It specifies the professional and personal characteristics required of the intervener; it also prescribes the behaviors or interactions to be exhibited by the intervener during the intervention delivery. Thus, the intervener characteristics become part of the intervention and present no threats to the intervention effects. In the SHIP example, the nature of the uncertainty management intervention demanded that the interveners have a background in oncology and psychosocial nursing and possess good communication or conversational skills to elicit information from the participants; this information is necessary for an accurate identification of the participants' concerns. Possession of these skills is a function of the interveners' professional characteristics, including their clinical training, and personal characteristics, including conversation and attentive listening abilities.

Despite the theoretical specification of characteristics required of the interveners, the actual characteristics possessed by the interveners may differ from the theoretical ones. For instance, the intervener may have the skill needed to carry the intervention but at a level different from that required for a successful implementation of the intervention. This is illustrated by the difference in the level of expertise between a novice and experienced clinician. Or the intervener may have other or additional personal characteristics that were not theoretically specified but that may influence or moderate the intervention effects. These extraneous intervener characteristics are discussed in this chapter as they affect the way in which the intervention is implemented and the participants' response to treatment.

Crits-Christoph and Mintz (1991) reanalyzed the data of 10 studies examining the outcomes of different types of psychotherapy (such as cognitive, behavioral, or dynamic) to determine the influence of the therapists on the outcomes of psychotherapy. In addition to the treatment factor, they represented the therapist ($N = 55$ across the studies, with each therapist assigned a code number) as a second factor in the analysis. The dependent variable was the averaged value on all the outcome measures included in each study. They analyzed the data collected across the studies with a two-way analysis of variance to examine the main and interactive effects of treatment and therapist. The therapist main effect was significant but moderate in some studies, accounting for 5%-10% of the variance in the averaged outcome measures. The therapist × treatment interaction effect was small in the majority of the studies, except one in which it accounted for 11% of the variance. These findings point to the potential confounding effect of the therapist. The authors concluded,

> Some modalities of treatment may be more prone to therapist effects (e.g., unstructured treatments like psychodynamic therapy may give more lee-way for aspects of the therapist to come into play, in contrast to highly structured treatments such as systematic desensitization or cognitive therapy . . .) . . . [and] the level of therapist experience may relate to the size of therapist effects, with less experienced therapists showing high therapist effects (near 50% of outcome variance) and highly experienced therapists showing no significant variability. Therapist variables such as competence or skill . . . have been shown to relate to outcome, and

Table 5.1 Influence of Intervener on Intervention Outcomes

A. Direct Effects
　　1. Manifestations
　　　Participants responding to the intervener rather than treatment
　　　Intervener expectancies or bias
　　2. Results
　　　Intervener and treatment effects confounded
　　　Incorrect conclusions

B. Indirect Effects
　　1. Manifestations
　　　Variability in implementation of intervention
　　2. Results
　　　Increased error variance
　　　Decreased statistical power to detect intervention effects

variability in these dimensions may explain the presence of therapist effects to some extent. Additionally, the processes used to select, train, and supervise therapists in a given study may be responsible for differences in the quality of therapists within a study. (pp. 23-24)

This study illustrates the influence of intervener characteristics on the effectiveness of an intervention in producing the intended outcomes. This influence can take two forms: direct and indirect effects on the expected outcomes (see Table 5.1).

Direct Effects of Interveners

The direct effects of the intervener on intervention outcomes is exemplified by participants reacting or responding to the behavior or attitude of the intervener rather than to the treatment itself. The nature of the interaction between intervener and participants depends on the personal and professional characteristics of the intervener and may have a direct effect on the participants' response to the intervention. For instance, overly friendly interveners may serve to increase social desirability bias that would be embedded in the participants' responses to the outcome measures. Thus, the success of the intervention may be related to the characteristics of the intervener or of the intervener-participant interaction and not necessarily to the nature of the intervention delivered.

The direct influence of the intervener's characteristics and of the intervener's interaction with the participants is becoming of interest to many researchers in the health care field. The success of health promotion programs relies on proper communication of information. Communication of a message is affected by the characteristic of the communicator: Interveners perceived as credible, sincere, and possessing characteristics similar to the audience are more likely to have an impact on the audience (Cooper & Croyle, 1984). The success of health programs for high-risk youth, including homeless and prostitute adolescent females, was found to depend not on the services provided but on the trusting relationships the public health nurses were able to establish with these vulnerable young women, who are often suspicious and lack trust (Deal, 1994). Similar conclusions were reached by Daro and McCurdy (1994), who reviewed the empirical literature pertinent to interventions for preventing child abuse and neglect: "A program's success often hinges on the qualifications and skills of its direct service providers. . . . Service providers must possess interpersonal skills desired for effective service provision, and overcome class and cultural barriers between provider and client" (pp. 410, 411). A supportive relationship between health care providers and clients was found to influence recovery in cardiac patients, with patients lacking the providers' support demonstrating lower scores on recovery, compared to others (Yates, 1995).

The intervener direct effect on the outcomes of an intervention can be also illustrated with the notion of experimenter expectancies and bias. Interveners are aware of their participation in a study and may alter the treatment in subtle ways so as to enhance or weaken its effects, depending on their belief in, level of interest in, and endorsement of the intervention. They could transmit their beliefs and attitudes to potential participants during recruitment or to participants receiving the treatment, through, say, their tone of voice or gestures. Thus, subjects may respond either favorably or unfavorably to the treatment based on the message communicated to them by the interveners. For example, interveners delivering a new treatment would be excited about it and motivated to prove that it is effective (Conrad & Conrad, 1994).

When this intervener effect (i.e., influence on response or bias or expectancies) occurs, the construct validity of the intervention is at stake since it will not be clear whether outcomes achievement is due to the intervention itself or to the expectations of the persons who deliver the intervention to participants (Cook & Campbell, 1979, p. 67). In this situation, the intervener effect confounds the intervention effects and acts as a threat to the conclusions' validity. This confounding effect is difficult, even impossible, to detect when the intervention is delivered by one person and is undoubtedly responsible, in part, for the frequent inability to reproduce the observed intervention effects in subsequent implementations of the intervention, under either experimental or real-life conditions (Bauman et al., 1994; Conrad & Conrad, 1994).

Indirect Effects of Interveners

The indirect effects of the intervener on intervention outcomes is represented by variability in the way the interveners implement the treatment in field settings that subsequently influences outcomes achievement. Individual differences in personal and professional characteristics influence the interveners' understanding of the essential features of the treatment to be delivered and their skills in carrying out the activities or procedures constituting the intervention. For example, case management is an intervention that could mean different things to different health practitioners. It may consist of any of the following: coordinating health-related services, providing social services, structuring the care of clients through a standardized care protocol that specifies which treatment should be given at what time for patients with a specific illness, planning the care of a patient based on identified individual needs, or involving the clients and their family in planning and implementing the care. Furthermore, interventions tailored to the needs of individual clients may require some procedural modifications; the form and extent of these modifications are influenced by the interveners' understanding of the intervention, specifically when the interveners are given minimal guidance or no protocol describing what exactly should be done in such situations. When the interveners interpret the intervention differently, the specific activities performed vary and deviate from the intervention as designed. Consequently, the intervention as delivered may not produce the intended outcomes.

Even if the interveners are provided with adequate explanation of the intervention, they may vary in the skills needed to perform the activities. Variability in skills can occur between different interveners involved in implementing the intervention or within the same intervener over time, for example, when his or her skills improve with repeated administration of the intervention. In turn, variability in the delivery of the intervention leads to variability in the achievement of outcomes. For instance, in the SHIP study, phone contacts were made with participants to identify their individual concerns and to provide appropriate counseling. The phone calls were made by two nurse-client managers with a background in psychosocial and cancer nursing. When the group of participants who received the phone contacts was compared to the control group, no significant differences were observed on the major outcomes, level of uncertainty, and self-care. But when the participants were divided into two subgroups associated with each of the nurse-client managers who made the phone contact, a significant difference in the outcomes was obtained between one of the subgroups and the control group, implying that there has been some variability in the way the intervention was delivered. Careful monitoring of the phone contacts made by the nurse-client managers revealed differences in the interveners' skills in communicating and relating with clients, which was an essential component of the intervention. One of the interveners displayed empathetic understanding to the participants, had refined communication skills, was very thorough and comprehensive in her assessment of the participants' concerns, and provided emotional support more frequently than the other intervener. This finding implies that the nurse-client managers' conversation and communication skills influenced treatment implementation and consequently outcome achievement.

Variability in treatment implementation leads to increased variance in the level of the outcomes achieved by individuals in the experimental group that is not attributable to the intervention. This within-group variance increases the error variance in tests of statistical significance, thereby decreasing statistical power to detect significant intervention effects.

Conventional Strategies for Dealing With Intervener Effects

In conventional experimental, outcomes-focused effectiveness research, the role of intervener characteristics has been neglected for several reasons. First, the intervention is usually implemented by a very small number of interveners, often only one, who is the researcher or a clinician, member of the research team. For instance, in studies evaluating the effectiveness of psychotherapy and psychoeducation, one or occasionally two therapists are asked to deliver the intervention (Crits-Christoph & Mintz, 1991; Devine, O'Connor, Cook, Wenk, & Curtin, 1988). With only one intervener, any potential intervener influence on the outcomes cannot be discerned since its effects are embedded in or confounded with the intervention effect. Second, it is usually assumed that all interveners are equal, having the same characteristics and minimal influence on the subjects, since they maintain objectivity and distance while providing the treatment. Therefore, it is assumed that the intervention is implemented in the same way across participants and that the intervener effect is constant across subjects.

Despite these assumptions, investigators use different strategies to eliminate or minimize any potential intervener effects, whether direct or indirect. First and foremost, researchers prepare an intervention protocol that provides background information on the intervention and its objectives, the specific activities to be performed, a detailed account of the procedures to be performed when implementing the intervention, and methods for dealing with any potential implementation problems. This protocol guides the researcher in identifying the skills required of the interveners, guides the training sessions, and guides the interveners in implementing the intervention as designed (i.e., maintains integrity of implementation in one study and across replication studies) or selecting appropriate alternatives when the intervention demands some judgment or decision on the part of the intervener. In the SHIP study, a standard teacher guide was prepared for each of the self-help classes. The teacher guide included the overall goal of the class session, the specific objective, the content to be covered, the activities to be performed in association with each objective, and the amount of time to be allotted to each activity. An assessment/appraisal/intervention protocol, derived from the intervention theory, was developed and followed during the UMI delivery. Providing the interveners with a protocol for delivering the intervention minimizes variability in its implementation and consequently the indirect effect of the intervener.

A second strategy to minimize potential intervener effects is to carefully select the interveners. Interveners who display the professional characteristics needed for a successful implementation of the intervention are usually selected. Possession of these skills is based on the intervener's discipline, education, training, and expertise in the field of interest. For instance, in the SHIP study the teachers who led the self-help classes had to have at least a bachelor's degree in a health-related field and some experience in working with patients with breast cancer. This experience

Table 5.2 Content of Intervener Training Sessions

---

1. Orientation to the research project
2. Explanation of the theory guiding the intervention
3. Discussion of the essential features of the intervention: What should be done, with
   whom, for what purpose, at what level, under what conditions, for how long, and how it
   should be done
4. Training in using any equipment required for delivering the intervention and in
   performing the activities constituting the intervention
5. Discussion of issues pertinent to the nature of the interpersonal aspect of the
   intervener-participant interaction
6. Presentation of strategies to address ethical and legal issues arising during the treatment
   phase or to decide on alternatives when facing potential implementation difficulties
7. Emphasis on following the intervention protocol across all subjects
8. Discussion of the issue of intervener effects

---

was necessary for the teachers to understand and attend to the needs of participants and to serve as a resource for them. In addition to technical skills, researchers tend to choose interveners who are highly motivated, credible, and reliable in their performance. Selecting interveners with specific personal characteristics that improve the delivery of the intervention is important for minimizing intervener indirect effects and for enhancing the internal validity of a study. But such a decision threatens the external validity of the findings, as these particular characteristics may not be present in the health care providers who would ultimately be responsible for delivering the intervention in their everyday practice (Conrad & Conrad, 1994; Kirchoff & Dille, 1994).

A third and equally important strategy is to provide intensive training sessions for the interveners. The content to be covered in a training session is summarized in Table 5.2. Some researchers advocate regular checks on the interveners' performance to monitor their adherence to the treatment protocol and solve any emerging problems. In the SHIP study, the class sessions were given by two teachers when possible, to maintain adherence to the teaching protocol; also, the class sessions as well as the uncertainty management intervention phone contacts were audiotaped to monitor and validate compliance with the intervention protocol.

The foregoing strategies minimize variability in the intervention implementation associated with intervener characteristics (i.e., the indirect effects). Little is written about strategies to reduce the confounding effects of the intervener, however, except for the double-blind procedure used in drug studies to counteract experimenter bias. This strategy is efficient in preventing bias in data collection, but it does not assist in ruling out or avoiding the direct effect of the intervener that confounds the intervention effects as described earlier.

Alternative Strategies for Dealing With Intervener Effects

The conventional strategies for dealing with intervener effects reduce variability in intervention implementation associated with the individual differences of the interveners. Therefore, they should be used in any intervention evaluation study. The alternative strategies proposed here aim at identifying, estimating, and even minimizing the direct and indirect effects of the intervener. Identifying and estimating the intervener effects and examining how they influence outcomes achievement are important to enhance not only the construct validity of the intervention and the internal validity of the study but also its external validity and applicability of the findings in the real world. In the real world, the intervention is delivered by numerous clinicians with various personal and professional characteristics. These natural differences among clinicians may be associated with variability in the implementation of the intervention and in the nature of the clinician-client interactions. Thus, it becomes essential to examine which and how the intervener characteristic(s) account(s) for this variability and to determine if the intervention is robust (i.e., it produces the desired effects) despite this variability in implementation. Results of such analysis address the clinical question, Who can deliver the intervention successfully?

The ability to answer this question requires the involvement of more than one intervener in delivering the intervention being evaluated. Multiple interveners vary in their personal and professional characteristics; this variability permits examination of the intervener effects on outcomes.

The strategy proposed to determine the intervener effect is borrowed from the psychotherapy literature. It consists of incorporating the intervener as a study variable, accounting for some of the variance in the outcomes. Using this strategy requires some modifications in the assumptions underlying effectiveness research: (a) individual differences in the interveners are acknowledged, since they reflect a naturally occurring phenomenon (the assumption of equality of interveners is rejected); and (b) the interveners are individuals interacting with the study participants (the nature and extent of this interaction vary across interveners and therefore might have an impact on the participants' response to the treatment). Thus, the impact of the intervener on the intervention outcomes must be examined.

Incorporating the intervener as a study variable can be accomplished with the following procedure. First, the characteristics required of an intervener to deliver the treatment are identified based on the intervention theory. These characteristics are then used as a basis for recruiting potential interveners. Whenever possible, a random sampling procedure is used to obtain a sample of interveners representing the population of interveners who would ultimately use the intervention (Bauman et al., 1994). The characteristics of the interveners should be reported, as is usually done for the study sample, so that potential users of the intervention would have an idea of who can implement it. The intervener profile can include, at least, age, gender, ethnicity, discipline, and educational background. Other characteristics of interest could be measured with standardized tests, such as health beliefs and attitudes.

Second, more than one intervener is included to deliver the same intervention. This is essential for identifying and estimating the extent of the intervener effects on the outcomes. When only one person delivers the same intervention to all participants, the intervener's potential effects are constant across the subjects and therefore cannot be identified or partialed out (Crits-Christoph & Mintz, 1991). Including more than one intervener introduces some variability that can be modeled and examined. There are two models for introducing the intervener-related variability: nested and crossed. In the nested model, different interveners are used in each treatment modality, and each provides the intervention to a group of participants. For instance, two interveners were assigned to make the phone calls in the uncertainty management intervention in the SHIP study; each was responsible for a group of participants. In the crossed model, each intervener provides all treatment modalities to all participants. This crossed design could be illustrated by having the same intervener make the phone calls and also lead the self-help classes.

Third, a record is kept of which intervener delivered which intervention to which participant. Keeping such a record is easier to accomplish when the intervention is delivered at the individual level, as in the case of the phone contact characterizing the uncertainty management intervention in the SHIP study. Maintaining a class attendance log in which participants and intervener present at each session record their names is an alternative strategy for maintaining such a record when the intervention is delivered at a group level. This recorded information is used to create a variable representing the intervener during data entry.

Fourth, the intervener variable is incorporated in the statistical analyses to determine the contribution of the intervener to outcomes achievement. Examining the intervener effects on outcomes consists of comparing the outcomes achieved by participants receiving the intervention that is delivered by the different interveners. The intervener is represented as a factor in an analysis of variance, that is, the intervener variable is considered a factor, either random or fixed, in addition to the treatment factor in a two-way analysis of variance. This analysis determines the treatment main effect, the intervener main effect, and the treatment × intervener interaction effect on the outcomes. Ignoring the intervener effect may result in biased estimates of the treatment main effect. It is important to use the correct error term, however; the *F*-ratio should be based on the model followed to represent the intervener to avoid Type I error when estimating the treatment effect. In the model in which the intervener is nested within treatments, to have significant treatment effects, the differences related to the treatment conditions should be greater than the differences related to interveners. Therefore, the correct error term for the *F*-ratio for the treatment main effect should be the between-intervener mean squares. In the model in which the intervener is crossed with treatments, significant treatment effects are contingent on the fact that the intervener is equally skillful in providing all the treatments. Thus, if an intervener is better at one treatment than at the other, then any observed difference between the treatments may be attributable to the intervener rather than to the treatment. Therefore, the correct error term for the treatment main effect *F*-ratio should be the treatment × intervener interaction term mean squares. These error terms take into account the nonindependence between the treatment and the intervener variables (Crits-Christoph & Mintz, 1991). When significant between-intervener differences are detected (i.e., the patients of some therapists tend to have better—or worse—outcomes than others), the analysis can be taken one step further: Between-intervener differences are explored in relation to individual interveners' personal and professional characteristics. The question to be addressed in this descriptive analysis is, What characteristic(s) is(are) responsible for the differences in the interveners' performance? This kind of knowledge is essential for the generalizability of findings in that it informs clinicians of the skills needed for a successful implementation of the intervention in everyday practice (i.e., it answers the question, Who would best fit to provide the intervention?).

The fifth step in the procedure to examine the interveners' effect consists of collecting data from the interveners pertinent to the activities they performed when delivering the intervention and to their perception of the dynamics of the intervention-delivery situation. Data on the interveners' perception of the dynamics involved in the treatment condition provide information about factors with the potential of interfering with treatment delivery or confounding the treatment effects. Interveners are asked to keep a diary or are interviewed by the researcher. They are encouraged to reflect on their behavior or interactional style with participants, to identify factors that facilitated or hindered the treatment delivery, and to recollect participants' responses to the intervention that are not captured by the standardized instruments measuring the outcomes of interest. These inherently qualitative data supplement the quantitative findings about the influence of the interveners' characteristics.

Last, qualitative interviews with participants are conducted to elicit information regarding their perception of the most effective aspect of the intervention. Specific questions about the intervener's personal and professional characteristics could be included. The participants' responses are then content-analyzed, and emerging themes are used to explain or validate the findings.

These strategies, if used in intervention evaluation studies, are effective in identifying the influence of the intervener characteristics on the outcomes and estimating the magnitude of their effects. As a result, statistical power is increased (since by including intervener as a variable accounting for some systematic variance in the outcomes, error variance is reduced) and the construct validity of the intervention is enhanced (since it becomes possible to disentangle the participants' response to treatment from their response to the intervener). Furthermore, with an improved understanding of which intervener characteristic contributes to a successful intervention implementation and how the intervener impacts the participants' response, generalizability or applicability of the findings to clinical practice is facilitated.

Setting Characteristics

The term *setting* refers to the environment in which the intervention is delivered. The environment selected for testing the intervention may be a controlled laboratory setting, a hospital unit, an organization or institution, a client home, a private office, a community clinic, or the community at large. Ignoring the potential influence of the setting on the outcomes expected of the intervention has serious implications for the external validity of conclusions. Just as the effects of intervener characteristics on outcomes cannot be identified until different interveners are included, so it is with the influence of the setting on outcomes. If the intervention is delivered in the same place, under the same conditions, across all participants, the setting is constant, and its effects are potentially confounded with the treatment effects. Thus, the setting is an aspect of the study that should be of concern in multisite field projects, since variability in the outcomes across the sites is a threat to the validity of conclusions regarding intervention effectiveness and therefore should be ruled out as a plausible alternative explanation of the findings.

Types of Settings

The setting, as a factor influencing the outcomes of an intervention, consists of the physical and psychosocial features of the environment in which the intervention is implemented. The physical features of interest in an effectiveness study include but are not limited to access or convenience of the setting location to participants; availability of equipment; the physical layout and its attractiveness in terms of noise level, ambient temperature, light, comfort of furniture, providing for privacy, and room interior design or decoration; familiarity to the participants; and general ambiance. The psychosocial features of the setting related to the social, political, economic, and geographic context of the study (Conrad & Conrad, 1994) include variables such as the organizational culture, norms and policies, standards and protocols of care, composition of an interdisciplinary health care team and differences in the skill mix in each group of providers, number of health care providers, and type of institution (Closs & Tierney, 1993; Finney & Moos, 1984; Tarlov et al., 1989).

Influence of Setting Characteristics

"The setting can mute or intensify effects depending on interactions with units [i.e., participants], treatments, and observations [i.e., measures of variables]" (Conrad & Conrad, 1994, p. 21). In a field experimental study with multiple sites, the site acts as a moderator of the treatment effects: It can facilitate or impede the implementation of the intervention and consequently the achievement of outcomes. Morse, Simon, Besch, and Walker (1995) reported on factors perceived by program staff as barriers to the conduct of a randomized clinical trial to evaluate community programs for patients with AIDS. Lack of clinic space, lack of financial resources, and lack of staff were considered as barriers influencing participant recruitment, retention, and compliance. Furthermore, those sites recruiting more participants had implemented clinic-based strategies such as flexible clinic hours, child care, and shelter and drug rehabilitation placement to enhance recruitment, retention, and compliance (RCC) efforts. Similarly, these same successful clinical sites had developed protocol-based strategies to enhance RRC by designing educational programs that explained clinical trial research to their primary care patients in a culturally sensitive yet simple way. In addition to affecting subjects' recruitment and retention, and sometimes attrition (Finney & Moos, 1984), the setting may impose some modification in the way the intervention is implemented. Hegyvary and Chamings (1975) examined the effects of preoperative instructions on the development of postoperative complications and on the use of analgesics. The results were not consistent across the two hospitals in which the study was conducted. Patients in one hospital required, on average, 4 days to return to a solid diet (compared to 3.4 days in the other hospital), requested more analgesics, and had a higher rate of postoperative infections than those in the other hospital. Differences in patients' initial status were ruled out as a source of variability in outcomes achievement. Differences in outcomes were related to variability in the clinical activities performed by the staff nurses in the two hospitals: Nurses were more involved in direct care than in nonclinical work in one of the two hospitals. This variability in nursing activities could explain the variability in treatment implementation: In the setting emphasizing nurses' involvement in direct care, staff nurses involved in patient preoperative education could have spent more time in this clinical activity, allowing them to attend to the patients' needs, and to present the information slowly and in detail.

Clinical experience and preliminary empirical evidence also suggest that the delivery of the intervention may vary across clinical settings. For instance, the type, frequency, and intensity of rehabilitation exercises that could be performed by clients differ when clients are institutionalized and when they are at home. In an institution, clients are scheduled to exercise on a regular basis under the supervision of a physical therapist, necessary equipment is readily available, and the exercises are rather well structured. The clients' situation at home may not be conducive to performing the exercises as prescribed. In a meta-analysis of studies evaluating the effectiveness of educational interventions on knowledge, self-care, metabolic control, and psychological outcomes in diabetic patients, Brown (1992) found that hospital-based educational programs produced larger effects for knowledge and metabolic control outcomes than outpatient clinics.

In summary, the characteristics of the setting affect the implementation of the intervention, which, in turn, affect the outcomes. The identification of the particular setting characteristic and the nature of its impact on outcome is based on the intervention theory guiding the effectiveness study.

Strategies for Dealing With Setting Effects

Strategies for dealing with the setting effects are very few, since the influence of the setting has been of little systematic interest. In the experimental tradition, any aspect of the environment that could affect the treatment-outcome causal connection is considered a nuisance or an extraneous factor contributing to the systematic variance that is not accounted for by the intervention. To minimize or eliminate the influence of these extraneous factors, investigators controlled aspects of the environment by holding them constant across subjects. For instance, when evaluating the effectiveness of sedative music in inducing relaxation, the researcher has to control for factors in the environment that influence relaxation. These factors include ambient temperature (uncomfortable temperature prevents subjects from relaxation), room light (bright light acts as a stimulant), noise level (loud noise startles subjects), and position assumed when listening to music (uncomfortable position is not conducive to relaxation). Researchers can control for these factors by adjusting the room temperature and maintaining it at the same level, by keeping dim light conditions, by using earphones to deliver the music, and by providing a soft recliner to all subjects. Such control is feasible in a laboratory setting. It is not easy, however, when the intervention is implemented under real-life conditions, especially in primary care settings, in which multiple factors are in operation and are not under the investigators' control. Alternative strategies for handling variability associated with the setting involves providing an adequate description of the setting(s), conducting the evaluation study in different settings, and incorporating setting as a variable in data analysis of a multisite clinical trial. The level of outcomes achieved and the causal relationship between the treatment and outcomes can be described within each setting as well as compared between the settings (Conrad & Conrad, 1994). Alternatively, a variable representing the different sites may be used as a factor in an analysis of variance or regression analysis, thus allowing one to determine and estimate the moderating effect of the setting on outcomes. This analysis and the interpretation of findings is similar to those described when examining the effect of the intervener.

In conclusion, the setting in which the treatment is delivered influences the way the intervention is implemented and consequently the expected outcomes. The effects of the setting cannot be identified under controlled experimental conditions and could confound the treatment effects. Conducting the evaluation study in different settings and incorporating setting as a factor in the analysis enhances the validity and the generalizability of the findings.

Summary

Examining the influence of the intervener and the setting on the outcomes expected of interventions improves the validity of conclusions regarding treatment effects. It also provides information to guide utilization of the intervention in clinical practice by specifying factors that facilitate or impede the intervention delivery and that are needed for yielding favorable outcomes. Despite these advantages, analyzing the intervener and setting effects should be guided by the intervention theory, which specifies whether or not the intervener and the setting have any significant influence on the outcomes, the particular characteristics of concern in a study, and the nature of their effects on outcomes achievement.

Chapter 6

INTERVENTION VARIABLES

For clinicians and investigators to provide interventions with predictable, favorable outcomes, they must (a) have a clear understanding of the presenting problem requiring resolution, (b) be able to select an intervention that is most appropriate for resolving the problem, (c) have an in-depth understanding of the processes through which the intervention resolves the problem or produces the desired outcomes, (d) be knowledgeable about the specific activities constituting the intervention and skillful in applying them, and (e) implement the intervention activities as originally designed and at the specified dosage. Briefly stated, clinicians and investigators require adequate understanding of the nature and rationale of the intervention to be provided and must deliver it as planned.

This chapter focuses on the aspects of the intervention that influence its effectiveness in achieving the intended outcomes. First, the characteristics of interventions are described and the issue of maintaining the integrity of intervention implementation in field settings is reviewed. Second, the conventional methods for monitoring integrity and for representing the intervention are examined and their limitations discussed. Last, alternative methods are presented, illustrated with examples from the SHIP study and pertinent literature.

Characteristics of Interventions

Interventions vary in their nature, their level of complexity, their dosage or strength, and the resources needed to carry them out. The diversity in these characteristics of interventions should be taken into consideration when planning and conducting a study for evaluating intervention effectiveness, as these characteristics have a direct impact on the integrity of intervention implementation, with a potential for erroneous conclusions.

Nature of Interventions

The nature of interventions is a characteristic that is derived and defined by the theory underlying the interventions. It is described in terms of the purpose for which the intervention is used, the rationale explaining the effects of the intervention, and the type of activities constituting the intervention. Understanding the nature of the intervention being evaluated facilitates the design of an effectiveness study. It directs the development of the intervention protocol, the implementation of the intervention, and the selection of outcomes variables and measures.

Purpose of Interventions

In general, nursing or health interventions and programs are designed and delivered to enhance the health status of clients. Some interventions aim at reducing the risk for an untoward condition, preventing the occurrence of a problem, or promoting healthy behaviors. For example, health education is planned to enhance the clients' awareness of risk factors, understanding of how the risk factors operate to cause illness, and repertoire of skills to minimize these factors. The ultimate outcome of these interventions is the absence of the undesired status. Other interventions aim at treating or resolving an identified health-related problem or a symptom experienced by clients. For instance, fluids with essential nutrients are given to restore body fluids lost during a surgical procedure. The intended outcome of these interventions is the resolution of the presenting problem. Still other interventions are designed and implemented to assist clients in managing the presenting problem or symptom or preventing complications associated with it. In this case, the problem or symptom cannot be resolved or cured for reasons such as lack of adequate understanding of its causative processes or unavailability of a proper remedy, and it may recur with debilitating consequences for the clients. For example, patients with pulmonary diseases experience dyspnea, which influences their physical and psychosocial functioning, and for which there is no definite remedy. Interventions are designed to alleviate this symptom when it occurs, such as slowing and regularizing breathing, and to assist clients in coping with its sequelae, such as performing relaxation to reduce apprehension and fear associated with dyspnea (Renfroe, 1988). The desired outcome is the proper management of the problem or symptom and the absence of complications. The distinction among interventions with different purposes is not meant to be exclusive. There are interventions with multiple purposes. For example, progressive muscle relaxation can be used to prevent and manage anxiety and to promote stress management and a sense of well- being.

As described above, interventions are used to prevent, resolve, or manage a health-related problem. Knowledge of a particular intervention's purpose guides the selection of an intervention to address the presenting problem appropriately and the identification of outcomes expected as a result of the intervention. The nature of the presenting problem determines the intervention to be used. For instance, a problem presenting as a *potential* problem (i.e., an identified inadequacy in the level of functioning with the potential of resulting in an actual problem) requires interventions that are aimed at preventing it or promoting health. An *actual* problem (i.e., a condition resulting from actual alterations in functioning) requires interventions aimed at resolving or managing it. A problem presenting as an actual alteration with the potential for complications may require an intervention with multiple purposes. Furthermore, client outcomes expected of interventions with different purposes vary. For instance, absence of the problem is an outcome expected of preventive interventions, resolution of the problem is an outcome expected of interventions with the purpose of treating the problem, and successful management of the problem and absence of complications are desired outcomes of interventions with the purpose of managing the problem. Differences in the expected outcomes have implications for outcomes selection and measurement. For example, resolution of the problem can be most appropriately measured with goal-attainment scaling methods, as described by Martin and Scheet (1992) and Inzer and Aspinal (1981).

Rationale of Interventions

Health interventions are rationally based, meaning that there is a reason or logical basis for the intervention. Interventions are applied in response to an identified problem. They are expected to initiate some processes intended to prevent, resolve, or manage the presenting problem or to achieve the desired outcomes. The processes may target the manifestations, level of severity of, or causative factors underlying the presenting problem. They are delineated by the intervention theory, which explains the why and the how of the intervention—that is, the intervention theory defines the problem for which the intervention is given, describes it, specifies its etiology, and elucidates the changes or chain of events that occur after the delivery of the intervention and that yield to the expected outcomes. The processes, as delineated by the intervention theory, determine how the intervention "works" in producing its intended effects or how it deals with the presenting problem (Chen, 1990). Thus, the mediating processes provide the rationale of the intervention. A rationale is a framework that "incorporates general orientations or models of the causes of problems, of tasks to be accomplished, and of the appropriate processes and outcomes of the intervention" (Adelman, 1986, p. 73). The rationale makes legitimate the use of the intervention to address the specific presenting problem.

For example, listening to slow tempo, soft music is an intervention used to relieve dyspnea. Slow tempo, soft music impacts dyspnea through two different processes. First, this type of music has a calm, relaxing effect on the body. Thus, it reduces anxiety, which is a factor often associated with or leading to dyspnea. Listening to soft music distracts the attention of the individual away from the stimulus producing anxiety by creating a mental imagery or a sense of pleasure or by serving as a second stimulus that suppresses the anxiety-provoking stimulus when both stimuli are received simultaneously by the thalamus (Soibelman, 1948). Second, slow tempo, soft music alters the respiratory pattern that characterizes dyspnea (i.e., its manifestation) through the following mechanism: The body's innate rhythms, such as the respiratory rhythm, are influenced by the rhythm and the tempo of the musical piece; thus, with music at a slow rhythm or tempo, the respiratory rhythm that is altered or increased when dyspnea is experienced is restored to normal. This example illustrates the point made earlier that interventions can target the manifestations or etiology of the presenting problem by initiating different processes mediating their effects.

Knowledge of the processes underlying the intervention assists in identifying the changes that occur as a result of the intervention, as specified by the intervention theory. When the theory describes these processes as changes in a series of variables mediating the relationship between the intervention and the intended outcomes, a causal model representing the linkages between the intervention, the mediating variables, and the outcomes is derived, as described in Chapter 3. The mediating variables can be measured and their hypothesized effects can be tested empirically.

Examining the effects of these mediating variables is essential for a valid interpretation of the observed outcomes: If the intervention fails to initiate the hypothesized processes, which are manifested by changes in the level of the identified mediating variables, then the intended outcomes will not be achieved as expected. Conversely, when the intended outcomes are achieved as expected, it is important to demonstrate that the outcomes are, in fact, linked to the hypothesized intervention processes. For example, health education aims at reducing the risk for cardiac diseases. It involves providing individuals with information about which factors increase the risk for cardiac diseases (such as smoking, high blood pressure, high fat intake, lack of exercise) and how these factors may cause cardiac diseases (e.g., high blood pressure leads to arteriosclerosis, which, in turn, reduces the blood supply to the heart) as well as instructions about strategies for reducing these risk factors (e.g., importance of a low sodium diet and how to prepare such a diet; importance of maintaining regular exercises and what type of exercises to perform, for how long, and how frequently). The intended outcome is a reduction in the level of the disease risk factors (such as decreased blood pressure). The hypothesized processes underlying health education are:

education → increased knowledge of risk factors and risk reduction
strategies → behavior, that is, application of the risk reduction
strategies → outcome, that is, reduced risk for or absence of cardiac
disease.

This model specifies that the link between education and reduced risk is mediated by knowledge and behavior, implying that the desired outcomes will not be achieved if the individuals did not understand the relationships between the risk factors and the occurrence of the disease, if they did not learn of strategies or behaviors for reducing risk factors, and if they did not actually use the strategies or modify their health-related behaviors.

Type of Intervention Activities

In addition to its purpose and rationale, the nature of the intervention is defined by the activities that comprise it. The activities are derived from the intervention theory. The theory specifies what should be done to produce the intended outcomes (i.e., the particular tasks or procedures) and how it should be done (i.e, the mode of delivery). For instance, Bulechek and McCloskey (1992) provided specific information about the activities constituting 336 direct care treatments that nurses perform. For each listed intervention, they provided the label and the definition of the intervention and the set of activities that nurses may perform to implement the intervention. Knowledge of the particular activities that should be performed to deliver the intervention assists in developing the intervention protocol. The protocol guides the interveners in implementing the intervention as designed and serves as a means for monitoring the integrity of the intervention implementation, as will be discussed later. Maintaining the integrity of the intervention or its consistent implementation across participants and settings in an effectiveness study is a prerequisite for a valid evaluation of its effectiveness (Carter, Moorehead, McCloskey, & Bulechek, 1995).

Level of Complexity

The level of complexity is another characteristic of the intervention. Level of complexity is a function of the type and number of activities the intervention comprises, as specified in the intervention theory. The activities of an intervention or the services of a program that are directed toward reaching some common objective form the components of the intervention or program (Bickman, 1985). For instance, psychoeducational interventions consist of two components: the psychological component, including activities such as support group, individual counseling, and encouraging ventilation of feelings, all aimed at enhancing psychological well-being; and the educational component, encompassing activities such as class discussion of a particular topic, provision of written materials, or demonstration of a particular skill, all aimed at increasing knowledge. The level of complexity varies from simple to complex. Relatively simple interventions or programs consist of one component formed of activities or services that do not require advanced skills for implementation. Examples of simple interventions that have been evaluated are using a cooling blanket to reduce body temperature (Caruso, Hadley, Shukla, Frame, & Khoury, 1992); sending prospective surgical patients a booklet including instructions for deep breathing, coughing, leg exercises, and ambulation, which are performed postoperatively to prevent complications (Rice & Johnson, 1984); and using nonoscillating waterbeds to maintain movement and increase the energy available for growth in premature infants admitted to a neonatal intensive care unit (Deiriggi, 1990). More complex interventions or programs consist of two or more components, composed of activities that require advanced skills for implementation. For example, Thackwray, Smith, Bodfish, and Meyers (1993) developed a complex intervention for treating bulimia nervosa. The intervention consisted of two components: The cognitive behavioral component included activities such as cognitive restructuring, problem-solving skill building, and assertiveness training. The behavioral component included activities such as self-monitoring of daily caloric intake and binge eating and purging and explaining the value of examining and changing environmental antecedents and behaviors. Wanich, Sullivan-Marx, Gottlieb, and Johnson (1992) developed a program for reducing the potential for delirium in hospitalized elderly. The program consisted of five components: (a) orientation and communication, (b) mobilization, (c) environmental modifications, (d) caregiver education, and (e) medication management.

The complexity of an intervention has implications for its implementation and evaluation. Successful implementation of complex, multicomponent interventions requires careful design and close monitoring of their delivery. A detailed protocol is needed to clarify the components of the intervention and to describe the specific activities or services forming each component, its mode of delivery, and its required dosage. The skills needed to carry out each component of the intervention have to be well specified, as they guide the selection of interveners. Complex, multicomponent interventions may require the selection of multiple interveners, each possessing the skills needed for delivering one or more components of the intervention. Having multiple interveners providing different intervention components demands (a) a careful design and coordination of how the components are delivered (i.e., the sequence of components to be delivered and the duration and frequency at which each is given), and (b) a careful monitoring of implementation to ensure that the components are delivered as designed. Evaluating complex, multicomponent interventions requires careful examination of the effects of the specific components, rather than the intervention as a package, on the outcomes. The components may influence the outcomes expected of the complex intervention in different ways; therefore, they can be studied separately.

Strength

For an intervention to be successful in resolving an identified problem, it should be strong enough to initiate the processes underlying its effects. Strong treatments contain large amounts of the ingredients leading to the intended changes; in contrast, weak treatments fall short of creating the expected changes or yield changes of small magnitude (Yeaton & Sechrest, 1981). The concept of strength of an intervention is very similar to the concept of dose of a medication. For instance, to be successful in treating a specific infection, the antibiotic should contain the ingredient that is most effective against the strain of bacteria causing the type of infection at hand. Giving penicillin to fight an infection caused by penicillin-resistant bacteria is inappropriate and will not produce the desired outcomes. Furthermore, the antibiotic should be prescribed and taken at the proper dose in order to be beneficial. The dose of an antibiotic refers to the amount, the frequency, and the duration for taking the medication. Failing to prescribe or take the antibiotic at the prescribed dose may result in unsuccessful treatment of the infection.

The strength (also called dosage) of an intervention refers to the a priori knowledge of the intensity and duration of the treatment needed to produce the expected changes (Sechrest et al., 1983). Intensity is represented by the amount of the activities that needs to be given and the frequency with which the activities are to be performed over a specified period of time. Duration refers to the total length of time the intervention is to be implemented for the expected effects to take place (Scott & Sechrest, 1989). Thus, the strength or dosage of an intervention is operationally defined by three dimensions: amount, frequency, and duration. An index can be developed based on these dimensions to represent the intervention strength. The following examples illustrate the strength of nonpharmacological interventions: (a) Progressive muscle relaxation: Participants are taught to tense their muscles as hard as possible for 15 seconds, then to relax them for 15 seconds (i.e., amount), over a period of 10 minutes; this relaxation exercise is to be performed twice a day (i.e., frequency) and as long as necessary (i.e., duration). (b) Patient education: The educational content related to management of symptoms associated with cancer treatment is covered in five group sessions; each session is expected to last 60 minutes (i.e., amount); one session will be given each week (i.e., frequency) for a total period of 5 weeks (i.e., duration); participants are expected to attend all five sessions to benefit from the intervention. (c) Uncertainty management intervention of the SHIP study: This intervention consisted of a semistructured phone interview that aimed at assessing the women's concerns and their uncertainty appraisal and providing appropriate interventions to relieve uncertainty. The length of the phone contact could vary depending on the women's willingness to express their concerns, the number of problems identified, and the number of interventions delivered. Thus, the length of the phone contact reflected the amount of activities given. One phone contact was scheduled for each week (i.e., frequency) and the women were encouraged to initiate the phone call if needed. The intervention was delivered over a 6-week period (i.e., duration). The strength of the intervention was represented by the sum of the length of phone contact across the total number of phone contacts made during the 6-week period.

The strength of an intervention can be identified through the intervention theory. The theory specifies the activities and their amount, frequency, and duration required to initiate the correct processes underlying the intervention effects (Sechrest et al., 1983). It is important to note that "some treatments are relatively fixed with respect to parameters of strength . . . [and that] for some treatments, virtually the only dimension of strength that can be varied is duration" (Yeaton & Sechrest, 1981, p. 158). The strength of the patient education intervention is relatively fixed in that all patients have to receive the same standard sessions for the same duration, whereas the only aspect of the strength of the progressive muscle relaxation that varies is the duration, which is left for the client to decide upon. The intervention theory determines which dimension(s) of strength is (are) fixed and which can vary.

Clinical experience and expertise may assist in determining the intervention strength needed to produce the desired outcomes. For example, an expert health educator can provide an estimate of the number and length of sessions needed for teaching patients certain topics. In field settings, the strength of an intervention is most likely to be determined by the patients' response to the treatment; if a patient responds more slowly than expected, the treatment intensity or duration is changed. For instance, a client with chronic obstructive pulmonary disease who attends a group session about strategies for managing dyspnea may experience difficulty carrying out these strategies. Individual sessions may be planned, during which the clinician reviews the information slowly, demonstrates the strategies, and clarifies points of special interest to the particular client. Individual sessions, in which the intervener and participant interact on an intensive, individual basis and the individual needs of the participant are met, may represent an intervention of higher strength than the group session.

Findings of previous studies evaluating the intervention effectiveness may provide information regarding the intervention dosage that produced the desired outcomes. Or these findings permit dose-response analyses that guide the selection of the strength of an intervention most appropriate for producing the desired outcomes. Howard, Kopta, Krause, and Orlinsky (1986) reviewed the psychotherapy literature supporting the conclusion that there is a positive relationship between the amount of psychotherapy and the level of patient benefit for the purpose of specifying the mathematical form of the dose-response relationship. They plotted the number of psychotherapy sessions to which the patients were exposed against the percentage of patients who improved within a certain number of sessions for each study they reviewed. They found that the dose-response functional relationships are quite consistent across studies. The functional relationships were described as a negatively accelerated curve. The function indicated that 10%-18% of the patients show some improvement before the first session of psychotherapy, 48%-58% show considerable improvement by the eighth session, 75% of patients improve by the end of 6 months of once-weekly sessions, and 85% by the end of a year of treatment. These findings imply that at least eight psychotherapy sessions are needed to achieve the intended outcomes in at least half of all patients.

Lacking any theoretical or empirical evidence to guide the determination of the appropriate dosage, the strength of an intervention can be determined by having experts (such as clinicians who developed the intervention or those who used it in their practice) rate it in terms of the level of change in outcome variables they would expect to occur. Yeaton and Sechrest (1981) requested experts to judge the strength of smoking modification treatments. The experts were given descriptions of the smoking modification treatments and asked to estimate the extent of change they would expect from these treatments. This study was based on the assumption that strong treatments result in large changes and weak treatments in small changes. An average correlation of .47 between the changes expected by the judges and the actual change in outcomes was obtained. The moderate correlation was attenuated by the reliability of the outcome measures, since in some instances the correlation was as high as .70. These findings indicate that the strength of an intervention can be determined a priori by expert clinicians.

Strength, defined in terms of the amount, frequency, and duration of a treatment, is an important intervention characteristic that determines the expected changes in the outcomes. Participants should receive the specified intervention strength to exhibit the intended outcomes. In field settings, participants may not receive the specified dosage and therefore they are less likely to achieve the desired outcomes. In this case, monitoring the intervention delivery, measuring the intervention strength actually received by the participants, and examining its association with the intended effects are necessary for valid interpretation of intervention effectiveness. Participants who do not receive the prescribed strength of an intervention are less likely to exhibit the intended outcomes. Therefore, knowledge of the intervention strength is necessary for valid interpretations of outcomes.

Resources

The success of a well-defined intervention is contingent on the availability of resources that are necessary for its appropriate implementation in the experimental or field setting. A proper delivery of an intervention requires inclusion of the full spectrum of target participants, selection of interveners with the skills needed for providing the intervention, availability of equipment or materials needed for performing the intervention activities, and organizational or institutional support for coordinating the intervention procedures. These resources represent the input factors needed for carrying out the intervention activities and have the potential to condition the implementation processes and the consequences of the intervention

(Chen, 1990; Lipsey, 1993). The presence of these resources facilitates the delivery of the intervention. The presence of some of these essential resources or their presence at a level less than required may result in variability in the way the intervention is delivered between participants and treatment situations, thus influencing the intervention effects (Rosen & Proctor, 1978).

The resources required for delivering an intervention are derived from the nature of the intervention and its level of complexity. The purpose and rationale of the intervention define the target participants who would most benefit from the intervention. The type of intervention and its activities determine the setting in which the intervention is to be delivered, the equipment or material needed for carrying out the activities, and the institutional support needed for organizing and coordinating the treatment operation. The intervention level of complexity specifies the skills required of the intervener to deliver the intervention properly. For instance, encouraging inpatients to listen to sedative music to alleviate anxiety requires (a) that potential participants accept the treatment, that is, they like to listen to music and the type of music provided; (b) a setting with minimal environmental noise, such as a private room; (c) the availability of tape players; and (d) staff support of the intervention, such as organizing the care activities to avoid interrupting the patient while listening to music.

A priori knowledge of which resources are needed is thus important to ensure their availability and consequently to facilitate the treatment implementation procedure. These resources form the conditions necessary for a successful delivery of the intervention and subsequent achievement of the intended outcomes.

Integrity

A priori knowledge of the intervention's nature, level of complexity, and strength and the resources needed for its implementation are essential for designing the intervention activities and planning strategies for its proper implementation in experimental or field settings. An intervention plan specifies what activities must be done and when, where, how, and by whom they should be carried out, thereby guiding the intervener in delivering the intervention. No plan, however, can ensure that the intervention is actually implemented as designed. Variability in treatment implementation affects its success in achieving the desired outcomes.

Integrity refers to the degree to which the treatment is delivered as planned (Yeaton & Sechrest, 1981). It reflects the discrepancy between what was initially planned and what is actually delivered. Lack of integrity in intervention implementation can be reflected in two ways. First is the deviation of what is implemented from what was intended for delivery, that is, the specific activities provided to participants differ from those originally designed. These deviations from the intervention as designed tend to occur in situations in which the intervention is not well defined or the interveners are not properly oriented. An intervention that is not well defined, specifically described, clearly circumscribed, and carefully operationalized is difficult to deliver since the specific activities to be performed are not well articulated and are open to different interpretations by the intervener(s) (Sechrest et al., 1983). Interveners who do not have a clear understanding of and guidance as to what activities to perform, when, and with whom will provide the intervention as they perceive it and not necessarily as designed. Different interpretations of the same intervention lead to implementation of activities that may not operationalize the intervention as intended. For instance, the intervention labeled "provide psychological support" may mean different things: listen to the client, encourage the clients to ventilate their feelings, or give positive feedback. Consider what the results would be if the intervener gave positive feedback instead of encouraging ventilation of feelings, as originally designed. The intended outcome of reduced emotional distress may not be achieved.

The second way in which lack of integrity occurs relates to participants being exposed to different components of the intervention, at different levels of strength. This kind of intersubject variability in the component and strength of the treatment received tends to occur when the intervention is not provided in a consistent or standardized manner across participants; when it is tailored to the individual needs of clients, so that each client receives different component and dosage (Rossi & Freeman, 1993); or when it requires the participants' active involvement in implementing the intervention in a community setting, away from the intervener's immediate supervision. For instance, cardiac patients are instructed to exercise on a regular basis. They may perform different types of exercises at home, with different intensity and duration, if their exercise program is not supervised by a health professional or is not well described to them; some choose to walk 2 miles, at their own pace, three times a week; others perform aerobic exercises for 20 minutes, daily; and still others prefer to use a stationary bicycle for 15 minutes, four times a week. These differences in the exercise performed result in variability in the strength of the intervention to which they are exposed and consequently in variability in the outcomes achieved. Differences in the level of outcomes achievement among participants in the experimental group leads to lack of significant treatment effects and potentially to incorrect conclusions about the effectiveness of the intervention (Rezmovic, 1984; Yeaton & Sechrest, 1981).

Integrity of an intervention implementation can be affected by several factors, such as ease of implementation of the intervention activities; the intervention level of complexity; adequacy of planning of operations (Yeaton & Sechrest, 1981); adequacy of description of and guidance for treatment practices; level of skill of the selected interveners (Rezmovic, 1984); level of staff and organizational commitment to the intervention (Sechrest et al., 1983); number of interveners and sites involved in its implementation; level of compliance of staff with the treatment protocol (Kirchoff & Dille, 1994); compliance of participants with the intervention protocol; adequacy of preparation and training of interveners; interactional style of interveners; and changes in organization policies that occur after the effectiveness study begins that have direct impact on the delivery of the intervention, such as changing the brand of equipment used or changing the composition of the nursing staff members who can provide the intervention being evaluated.

In summary, when implementing an intervention in experimental or field settings, several factors inherent in intervention activities and re-sources needed for carrying them out influence the way it is actually delivered, leading to a discrepancy between what was planned and what was actually delivered. Lack of intervention integrity threatens the validity of conclusions about treatment effectiveness:

> To correctly attribute the observed outcomes of a social program to the intervention, the researcher should have empirical evidence on the extent to which program components were implemented. Without such evidence, researchers may erroneously conclude that an intervention was ineffective when, in fact, treatment implementation was inadequate to afford a valid test of the program. (Scheirer & Rezmovic, 1983, p. 599)

Reaching erroneous conclusions about the effectiveness of an intervention that has not been appropriately implemented has been referred to as committing Type III error (Basch & Gold, 1986; Hoefer, 1994).

Conventional Strategies for Dealing With Type III Error

Laboratory Experiments

In a pure experimental study conducted in the controlled setting of a laboratory, the chances of committing Type III error are minimal, due to the control exerted by the researcher over the experimental condition. Traditionally, the investigator is in command of the laboratory situation and regulates the treatment operations. The experimenter develops the treatment protocol that describes the nature and the strength of the treatment, specifies the sequence of the activities to be performed, and provides the details of the procedures to be carried out. The treatment protocol is applied in a standard way across all subjects assigned to the experimental group. The interveners are selected carefully and trained intensively in the intervention procedures. Furthermore, they are required to maintain objectivity when interacting with subjects to avoid any potential influence on the subjects' response to treatment. The setting is arranged in a way that facilitates the delivery of the intervention. The equipment needed for the intervention activities is readily available and constantly checked for proper functioning, the environmental factors that could influence the treatment effects are controlled for, and the organizational or institutional influence on the experimental operations is often minimal. The treatment implementation is under full control of the experimenter; he or she determines who gets the treatment and who does not. This ensures that the subjects in the control group are not accidentally exposed to the treatment. The experimenter also determines what is given to the subjects in the experimental group, at what level, when, where, how, and by whom, thus ensuring that the subjects in the experimental group are exposed to the same treatment, at the same strength, and in a manner consistent across all subjects. The delivery of the treatment, which is periodically checked, and the control of the experimental conditions enhance the consistency in treatment delivery across subjects.

Controlled laboratory conditions make it relatively easy to deliver the treatment as planned, in a uniform manner, in the right amount, to the right subjects, at the right time (Lipsey, 1990). This uniform treatment implementation justifies the traditional method for measuring and representing the treatment in the statistical analyses of an experimental study. The treatment is usually measured as a dichotomy that reflects the subjects' experimental group membership (represented as 1 for the control group and 2 for the experimental group). This dichotomous treatment variable is then used to represent the independent variable in an analysis of variance. In the statistical model of an analysis of variance, the intervention effects show up as a change of a constant value in each subject's score on the outcome variable. The constant value could be either negative or positive, depending on the hypothesized treatment effects. For example, relaxation exercises might be expected to reduce high blood pressure, demonstrated in a reduction (i.e., a negative value) of, say, 30 mmHg in the posttest blood pressure of subjects in the experimental group. In contrast, relaxation exercises enhance the sense of well-being, manifested by an addition (i.e., a positive value) of, say, 10 points to the experimental subjects' posttest scores on the Index of Well-Being. In both situations, subjects in the control group are not expected to show any change in their posttest outcome scores. The constant values added or subtracted from the experimental subjects' scores represent the differences between the treatment and the control groups. This representation of the treatment variable "implies that each subject in the treatment condition receives the same dose of treatment and each subject in the control condition receives the same non-dose. It also implies that with a given treatment dose each subject responds with the same effect" (Lipsey, 1990, p. 158).

Field Experiments

Maintaining a uniform treatment implementation is possible under controlled experimental conditions and when the intervention activities and strength are fixed across subjects, but integrity and uniformity of treatment delivery cannot always be sustained in real-world field experiments, in which the researcher has minimal control over the experimental conditions. A researcher conducting an intervention effectiveness study in the real-world setting may elicit the assistance of staff in recruiting target participants, entrust the delivery of the intervention to various clinicians, and select different sites for conducting the study. Variability in these experimental elements results in variability in the delivery of the intervention. Thus, the assumption of uniform treatment implementation is challenged: "The non-uniformity of service delivery and service receipt across program implementation sites and, within sites, across program participants is becoming widely recognized" (Cook & Poole, 1982, pp. 425-426). Lack of treatment integrity becomes an acute problem in situations in which (a) the treatment is complex, involving several components that are applied differentially based on individual client needs; (b) some or all intervention activities are to be carried out by the participants, under minimal supervision from the intervener; and (c) the treatment is found beneficial and some form of it is delivered to the subjects in the control group (Lipsey, 1990).

When the treatment delivered deviates from the planned treatment, the processes underlying its expected effects are not initiated. Therefore, the outcomes expected from the treatment as planned are not achieved (Rossi & Freeman, 1993), resulting in Type III error. When experimental participants actually receive different types or doses of the treatment, the within-experimental group variance in the outcome variable increases. With variability in the type and dose of the treatment received, the amount of change in the outcome variable scores is not constant across the experimental participants: For some it will be low, and for others it will be high, taking either a positive or a negative value. This individual variability in the level of outcome achieved increases the error term (i.e., the within-group variance) of statistical tests and reduces the sensitivity to detect significant group differences (Lipsey, 1990). When participants in the control group are exposed to a similar treatment or to a low dose of the treatment offered to participants in the experimental group, all participants show some amount of change in the outcome variable, thus minimizing any difference between the means of the experimental and control groups. The result is a decreased power to detect treatment effects (Shapiro, 1984). It is important to note here that the selection of a control group influences the contrast between the treatment and the control group means. If the control condition chosen does not differ much from the treatment condition, the contrast between the group means is diminished. For instance, if the treatment as usual (i.e., standard care) incorporates some component(s) of the treatment being evaluated and is selected as the control condition, the contrast between the groups is reduced. Similarly, placebo conditions are some-times quite similar to the treatment conditions for which they serve as controls; thus, the contrast is decreased, manifested by nonsignificant differences between the groups (Lipsey, 1990).

The traditional strategies suggested to reduce Type III error in field experiments are similar to those used in laboratory settings. They include (a) developing a protocol, (b) training the interveners, (c) requesting the interveners to follow the protocol when implementing the intervention, (d) checking periodically the actual delivery of the intervention by the various interveners in various sites, and (e) pilot-testing the intervention to deter-mine its feasibility and recognize and resolve problems prior to its actual implementation in the field. Although these strategies improve the integrity of treatment implementation, they do not assess or examine what was actually delivered to each participant and at what dose or whether the hypothesized processes underlying the intervention effects took place. Such an analysis provides an accurate description of the intervention implemented, determines the intervention strength associated with the most benefit to clients, enhances the understanding of how the intervention works, and consequently improves the validity of the conclusions regarding intervention effectiveness. Therefore, alternative strategies that permit analyses of the effects of the intervention as delivered are needed.

Alternative Strategies for Dealing With Type III Error: Process Evaluation

Alternative strategies for dealing with Type III error were devised in response to the concerns arising from the use of the conventional, out-comes-focused approach in effectiveness research. These concerns can be summarized as the lack of adequate information about the theoretical model guiding the design of the intervention and explaining its effects (Marfo & Dinero, 1993; Mullen, Mains, & Velez, 1992; Simmons-Morton, Mullen, Mains, Tabak, & Green, 1992; Shonkoff et al., 1988) and about the type and strength of the intervention components received (Daro & McCurdy, 1994; Marfo & Dinero, 1993; Moskowitz, 1993). The absence of data about the implementation of and the processes underlying an intervention hampers the interpretation of outcomes evaluation results (Rossi & Wright, 1984). When an intervention is found to be ineffective, such data can help inform whether the observed outcomes are attributable to inadequate intervention implementation, design, or theory (Moskowitz, 1993). When the intervention is found to be effective, such data are invaluable in validly attributing the outcomes to the intervention, in understanding how the intervention or its components work(s) and under what conditions and for which type and level of severity of the presenting problem, in identifying the intensity and duration at which the intervention is most effective, and in learning about the specific manner in which it is best delivered. Therefore, it is recommended that the evaluation of an intervention should address not only the question of whether the intervention worked, but why it worked or failed to work.

Definition of
Process Evaluation

Process evaluation is a strategy for addressing the questions of why and how the intervention works. Process evaluation involves the measurement of what was actually done during the intervention implementation to effect the intended changes (Reid & Hanrahan, 1988). It encompasses a variety of data collection activities aimed at monitoring the integrity of implementation and at examining the processes mediating its effects (Dignan, Michielutte, Sharp, Young, & Daniels, 1991). Process evaluation is concerned with the degree of implementation, the implementation processes, and the mediating processes (Halvorson, Cohen, Brekke, McClatchey, & Cohen, 1993; Judd & Kenny, 1981; Scheirer & Rezmovic, 1983).

Monitoring the degree of implementation involves assessing the extent to which the intervention was implemented as planned. It covers three aspects. The first is *the extent to which full participation* by the target population was achieved: Who made up the target population? How many participants were recruited? How many refused the treatment? What were the reasons for refusal? What are the characteristics of those who accepted versus those who refused the treatment? How do they compare to the target population? The second aspect is *the intervention characteristics* as specified in the intervention theory, including its purpose, its components, and its strength. The third aspect is *the intervention in use,* or as actually delivered to the participants: Was the intervention delivered at all? Are the intervention activities consistent with those initially planned? What intervention component(s) was (were) received by each participant? At what intensity and for how long? Were the intervention components delivered in a standard manner to all participants? (King, Morris, & Fitz-Gibbon, 1987; Rossi & Freeman, 1993). Briefly, monitoring the degree of implementation provides data about who received what intervention component, at what dose, and how.

Evaluating the implementation processes consists of documenting the changes that were needed or made for successfully implementing the intervention. Data on implementation processes provide for (a) *a description of the setting(s)* in which the intervention was implemented (What kind of setting was used? How many sites were selected for implementation? What are the characteristics of these sites in terms of the physical layout, the staff, and the organizational support? Was the staff involved in any aspect of the study? What administrative arrangements were necessary to facilitate the intervention implementation? Did any event that might affect treatment implementation occur during the study period, such as the introduction of a new treatment protocol?), (b) *an account of the equipment* used to deliver the intervention (What type of equipment was required for performing the intervention activities? Was the same type of equipment used across participants?), and (c) *a description of the interveners* delivering the intervention (What are their professional and personal characteristics? Were they subjected to training sessions? What was covered during the training sessions? [King et al., 1987] How many interveners were included? How did they handle participants? Were participants nested or crossed across interveners?). Briefly, evaluating the implementation processes provides data about contextual factors that are necessary for a successful delivery of the intervention.

Analyzing the mediating processes includes two steps. The first consists of *identifying the causal chain* linking the intervention to the outcome variables. The causal chain explains how the treatment works; it specifies the mechanisms through which the intervention is expected to produce its effects. These mechanisms represent the structural transformations that the intervention brings about and that result in the intended outcomes (Chen, 1990; Lipsey, 1993). The structural transformations are reflected by changes in key variables that mediate the expected treatment effects. Therefore, if the treatment fails to initiate the mediating processes, the treatment will not exert any effect on the outcomes (Judd & Kenny, 1981).

The second step involves measuring the identified mediating variables. Their *relationships to the treatment variables and to the outcomes* are analyzed empirically, using appropriate statistical tests. This analysis determines whether or not the treatment was successful in initiating the hypothesized processes and consequently the expected outcomes.

In summary, process evaluation is a strategy for collecting data on the actual intervention received by the clients, on the resources needed for delivering the intervention, and on the processes that mediated the effects of the intervention. Information about the implementation of the intervention and about its theoretical underpinnings are necessary for an accurate interpretation and valid conclusions regarding the effectiveness of an intervention.

Selection of Methods for Process Data Collection

Process data can be obtained by reviewing documents and through observation, surveys or questionnaires, or interviews, using quantitative or qualitative data collection approaches. The advantages and disadvantages of these techniques are presented in Table 6.1.

The selection of a specific method for collecting process data is guided by a variety of factors, including but not limited to availability of resources that facilitate the use of the method, such as availability of equipment, time, cost, transportation, and trained interviewers or observers; acceptability of the method to potential respondents; burden imposed on the research or clinical staff and participants, with the potential for obtaining incomplete data; and the method's level of intrusiveness and potential of violating the ethical principles of privacy, confidentiality, and anonymity. Most important, the selection of a method for collecting process data is determined by the nature of the data to be gathered. The nature of the data reflects the conceptual and operational definitions of the process variable(s) of interest.

The next section presents methods for obtaining data pertinent to the degree of implementation, the implementation processes, and the mediating processes underlying interventions.

Degree of Implementation

The degree of implementation is reflected by coverage, characteristics of the intervention, and intervention in use.

Table 6.1 Advantages and Disadvantages of Methods for Collecting Process Data

Method	Advantage	Disadvantage
Existing documents	inexpensive readily available	incomplete information questionable validity and reliability
Setup documents	tailored to the evaluation project at hand	inconsistency in data recording burden on respondents

Observation	assessment of nonverbal
	    cues during intervention
	    or interaction
		requires intensive training
		expensive
		time consuming
		influences the behavior of those
		    being observed (reactive)

Questionnaire/
    survey
	inexpensive
	reaches a large number
	    of participants
		potential for biased responses
		potential for incomplete data
		potential for misunderstanding
		    item content or response option

Individual interview	well accepted complete data with clarification assessment of nonverbal cues reaches illiterates	expensive time consuming potential for biased responses potential for interviewer bias

Focus group	rapid collection of data at
	    less cost (compared to
	    individual interview)
	opportunity for clarification
	opportunity to examine
	    group process
		small number of participants
		potential for moderator bias
		potential for domination of group
		    discussion by some participants
		potential for peer pressure

Coverage. The extent to which potential participants are reached can be obtained through reviewing the research project or clinical or field-setting activity log. The research project activity log provides information about the sites selected for recruitment, the number of target participants recruited, the number who consented or refused to participate, the number assigned to the experimental and control groups, the number excluded from the study, the number who dropped out at each point of data collection if a repeated-measures design was used, and the reported reasons for refusal or dropping out of the study. The clinical or field-setting activity log provides information about the number of clients seen at the clinic, the health care provider who took care of the client, the presenting complaint or problem, and the treatment given. When a program targets the community at large, Rossi and Freeman (1993) suggest conducting a survey of target participants to inquire about their awareness of the intervention or program, their level of participation, the reasons for nonparticipation, and their standing on some characteristics of interest. For example, in an attempt to reduce inappropriate utilization of emergency room services, a group of community hospitals located in a large metropolitan area developed a pamphlet instructing the public on what types of conditions are considered urgent, requiring emergency medical attention, and which ones can be handled by walk-in clinics or general practitioners. The pamphlet was made available to the public in hospital emergency departments; community, hospital, and private clinics; drug stores; and grocery stores. The community at large was surveyed to determine the extent to which the pamphlet was actually picked up and read by the targets (i.e., the extent to which the intervention reached the target population) (A. M. Green, personal communication, September 1995).

Characteristics of intervention. The intervention theory delineates the characteristics of the intervention and the processes underlying its effects. In the absence of a well-defined theory, the effectiveness study proposal and the protocol guiding the intervention delivery can be reviewed thoroughly to identify the theoretical framework guiding the intervention, the specific purposes of the intervention; its components and strength; the key mediating variables and their conceptual and operational definitions; and the hypothesized linkages between the intervention, mediating variables, and expected outcomes. This information provides for a description of the intervention as planned, which is used as a reference for examining the integrity of implementation and guides the design of the evaluation study and the selection or development of the tools to measure the intervention characteristics, mediating variables, and outcomes, as well as the statistical analyses. Alternatively, when written information about the intervention characteristics is not available, clinicians or staff members involved in delivering the program may be surveyed and interviewed. The survey or interview aims at identifying the activities or services offered, the rationale for them, and the intensity and duration of these services, as perceived by clinicians. Focus-group sessions could also be conducted to gather similar data or to reach a consensus on the key characteristics of the intervention.

Responses may be content-analyzed to provide a description of the program components, strength, and underlying processes.

Intervention in use. Data pertinent to the actual delivery of the intervention can be obtained by different methods. An intervention activity log can be set up by the investigator, in which interveners can record which activity was performed for what patient, at what time, at what dosage, and for how long. For instance, in the SHIP study, an attendance log was kept for the self-help classes; in it the class leaders recorded the date and time of each class offered, the names of the women who attended each class session, and whether or not the women initiated an individual contact with the class leader requesting additional information.

The interveners can be asked to maintain field notes of problems encountered during implementation or comments made by the participants about the intervention. For example, in a pilot study examining the feasibility and acceptance of music as an intervention to relieve dyspnea, the research assistants were asked to write down any comments made by the participants about the ease of using music or about their impression of the intervention. In fact, some patients said that listening to music was helpful in relieving dyspnea but wondered whether it was the music or the mere fact of stopping activity and sitting in a chair (which they were asked to do while listening to music) that was actually responsible for relieving dyspnea (McBride, Graydon, & Sidani, 1996). These participants' comments have important implications regarding the mechanisms explaining the effects of listening to music on dyspnea.

The actual delivery of the intervention can be monitored through observation of the activities performed by the intervener or the participant, if possible. Observation is useful (a) in determining the extent to which the intervention activities are performed as planned (e.g., the observer is given a checklist derived from the intervention protocol, incorporating the steps for, say, flushing an intravenous line with saline; observes the intervener performing the procedure; and rates the extent to which each step was carried out as specified in the checklist), (b) in examining the interactional and behavioral style of the intervener and the participants (e.g., an observer can attend the class discussion and note the participants' reactions and behaviors) (King et al., 1987), and (c) in exploring the operations constituting a complex, multicomponent intervention or program for which components are not well described a priori.

In situations in which the actual implementation of the intervention cannot be observed directly for reasons related to invasion of privacy, logistics, and intrusiveness, diaries can be used. Interveners and participants may be requested to report on the intervention activities they performed and at what dosage. Similar information can be obtained by interviewing or surveying interveners and participants or by reviewing the clients' medical records (Dignan et al., 1991). For example, Archbold et al. (1995) evaluated a program designed to increase the preparedness and competence of family members providing long-term care for frail elders. As a means for monitoring the delivery of the program services, they recorded the number of home visits made to the experimental participants, the number of phone calls received from participants, and the type and number of strategies tried for each presenting problem. These kinds of data capture not only the components of the intervention actually delivered to participants but also the strength at which it was given.

Implementation Processes

The implementation processes are described in terms of the setting, material, and interveners involved in delivering the intervention.

Description of setting. Structured or semistructured observation is the most useful method for describing the actual setting in which the intervention was delivered. It provides data about the physical layout and the social environment of the site. A list of environmental elements to be observed, derived from the intervention theory, can guide data collection. Reviewing the minutes of research staff and intervener meetings can provide information about the administrative arrangements that were made to facilitate the implementation process, the problems encountered during the implementation, and the events that took place during the implementation period and that might influence the effectiveness of the intervention in producing the desired outcomes (Halverson et al., 1993). For example, when the introduction of multiskilled workers is evaluated in terms of its impact on patient outcomes, reviewing the minutes of administrative and in-service meetings held with the staff to introduce the change provides information about the social climate prevalent at the time. The staff reaction to the change may jeopardize the integrity of implementation of the change and consequently the achievement of expected outcomes.

Account of material. Information about the type of material needed for delivering the intervention (such as audiovisual equipment for patient education) can be obtained by reviewing the intervention theory or protocol. Data about the material actually used when delivering the intervention could be gathered through observation or through interviewing or surveying the interveners.

Description of interveners. Information about the skills required of the interveners can be gathered from the intervention theory, the description of their roles and responsibilities, and the training-session plan. The actual skills possessed by each intervener involved in the study implementation can be assessed toward the end of the training session or during the implementation phase by testing or by observing them while actually delivering the intervention. Other professional and personal characteristics of the interveners may be assessed by interviewing or surveying the interveners, using well-developed instruments when possible. For example, in a small-scale study aimed at exploring sources of variability in the care provided to cognitively impaired elderly persons, the nurses' level of knowledge about the standards of care and the nurses' attitude toward cognitive impairment were considered factors with direct impact on the care provided and consequently on the patients' outcomes. The nurses' knowledge was measured with case studies presenting commonly encountered clinical situations to which the nurses responded by developing a plan of care to resolve the identified problems. The nurses' attitudes were measured with an established instrument, the Custodial Mental Health Scale (K. McGilton, personal communication, February 1996).

Mediating Processes

The key mediating variables and their hypothesized relationships to the intervention and its outcomes are identified by reviewing the intervention theory explaining the intervention effects. When the processes mediating the intervention effects are not explicitly stated a priori, the researchers or clinicians responsible for developing or implementing the intervention are interviewed, individually or in a group, or surveyed. The purpose of the interview or survey is to inquire about the researchers' perception of how the intervention works. Qualitative methods for data collection and analysis are helpful in exploring and mapping the complex links between the processes underlying the intervention and the outcomes (Chen, 1994; Reid & Hanrahan, 1988; Steckler, Eng, & Goodman, 1991). For example, in the SHIP study described in the first chapter, the interventions were informed by two complementary theories proposing that the effects of the interventions (including the self-help classes, the independent study, and the uncertainty management intervention) on adjustment to breast cancer and its treatment are mediated by appraisal of the situation by the women as a challenge or a threat, by their enabling skills, and by their success in managing uncertainty. The three mediating variables were measured with established scales, and their effects on the outcome were tested empirically.

In addition to these theoretically prespecified variables, variables reflecting the participants' reactions to the intervention may interfere with or mediate the success of the intervention in producing the desired outcomes. Examples of such variables include the participants' understanding of the intervention, their perception of the utility and ease of use of the intervention, and their level of satisfaction with its components (Dignan et al., 1991; Halverson et al., 1993). Crano and Messe's (1985) study illustrates the influence of participants' comprehension or knowledge of the treatment on the expected outcomes. The intervention consisted of varying the cost of electricity to consumers as a function of the time of day at which it was used, so that the cost of electric power was higher during peak hours than at other times. Consumers were informed of the variations in cost in a letter sent to the households assigned to this experimental condition. The consumers' comprehension of the billing procedure was measured. Results of the study indicated that the time-of-use billing procedure had little, if any, impact on electric usage; rather, the level of comprehension had a direct, significant effect on the outcome. In the SHIP study, the participants' perception of the helpfulness of the self-help classes' activities were measured by an investigator-developed tool. Participants were asked to rate how helpful each activity was to them on a three-point scale ranging from 1 (*Didn't help*) to 3 (*Helped a lot*). The perceived level of helpfulness had significant effect on the women's adjustment to their illness; in particular, women who perceived the classes as helpful showed a gradual improvement in their ability for self-care (Sidani, 1994). This finding implies that perceived helpfulness of the content covered in the classes is a variable mediating the intervention effects on self-care abilities—that is, to be effective in enhancing self-care abilities, the content covered in the class should be perceived as helpful to the women.

In summary, the selection of a method for gathering process data is guided primarily by the nature of the variables used to operationalize the processes mediating the intervention effects and the degree of implementation. The selection of a method should consider the extent of bias inherent in each individual method:

> When examining a complex construct such as degree of implementation, the use of multiple techniques is desirable to avoid the method specific biases associated with each individual technique. The larger the number and variety of implementation measures used, the greater the likelihood that method-specific biases will be detectable, that multiple components of the innovation will be examined, and that implementation, therefore, can be validly assessed. (Scheirer & Rezmovic, 1983, p. 610)

Finally, the selection of specific measures should be based on their reliability and validity; the congruence between the content of the measure and the operational definition of the variable should be carefully assessed to improve construct validity (Scheirer & Rezmovic, 1983; Trochim, 1985).

Process Analysis

The data gathered on the intervention processes are not useful until appropriately analyzed. The analyses are done for descriptive, comparative, and evaluative purposes.

Description. Adequate description of the intervention and its implementation is essential for understanding, disseminating, replicating, or utilizing it in various clinical settings. The description incorporates information about the intervention as planned and as delivered, including its components and their strength, the clients who accepted or refused to participate, the participants who dropped out, the setting for implementation, the material required for carrying out the intervention, the characteristics of the interveners, and the reaction of participants to the services delivered. The description is either qualitative, presenting narrative accounts of the implementation, or quantitative, presenting the data graphically or numerically (Rossi & Freeman, 1993). The use of a qualitative or quantitative approach to describe the intervention as delivered is determined by the extent to which the intervention and mediating variables were defined, conceptually and operationally, a priori, and monitored and measured.

Comparison. Two types of comparison are made when analyzing process data. The first compares the intervention as delivered to the intervention as planned, in order to examine the integrity of the intervention. Assessing the extent to which the implemented intervention deviates from or conforms to the designed intervention determines the appropriateness of evaluating the effectiveness of the intervention in achieving the desired outcomes: An intervention that was drastically modified during implementation or that was not implemented at all cannot be expected to produce the expected changes (Rossi & Freeman, 1993). This comparison is basically analytical, involving mapping the characteristics of the intervention as planned, summarizing the data gathered on each characteristic during implementation, and assessing the correspondence between the two (Trochim, 1985).

The second type of comparison is concerned with differences between participants and nonparticipants and differences in implementation between settings and interveners, if more than one of each were used. Comparing clients who accepted the treatment to those who refused, on demographic characteristics and other personal attributes if possible, provides information on the extent of target population coverage, the extent of acceptability of the intervention by potential clients, and the population to which the findings can be generalized. Comparing participants who stayed to those who dropped out offers some clues as to who would be most compliant with the treatment, how to improve the intervention and its delivery to fit the demands of different client subgroups, and what strategies could enhance compliance with treatment. Examining differences in treatment implementation across settings and interveners provides information about the resources needed for an optimal or successful implementation of the intervention (Rossi & Freeman, 1993). If differences in the type and strength of the intervention received by participants exist between settings or interveners, they should be accounted for when evaluating the impact of the intervention on outcomes. Accounting for the differences related to the intervener and the setting, as described in Chapter 5, increases the sensitivity to detect significant effects and conditions under which the intervention is most effective.

Evaluation. In an evaluative analysis, the effects of intervention as delivered, rather than as planned, and the effects of the mediating variables on the expected outcomes are examined empirically. The components of the intervention actually received by the participants and the dosage at which they were received are used to reflect the intervention in the statistical analyses, rather than the traditional dichotomy representing group membership (i.e., intention-to-treat analysis). The dosage of the intervention or its components is measured on all participants using a predetermined scale. The lowest value on this scale is 0, indicating non-exposure to any dose of the intervention. Participants in the experimental group are assigned values on this scale that represent the different doses of the intervention or its components that they actually received. For instance, in a study conducted to examine the association between participation in an outpatient cardiac rehabilitation program and psycho-behavioral outcomes, Conn, Taylor, and Casey (1992) measured the level of participation in the rehabilitation program by the number of sessions attended by each participant. Results of correlational analyses indicated that with increased participation subjects reported better health; increased self-esteem, quality of life, engagement in exercise, and compliance with diet and medication regimen; and decreased anxiety and depression. Similarly, Condelli and Hubbard (1994) examined the relationship between the time spent in drug treatment and outcomes of clients in therapeutic communities. Logistic regression analysis showed that the longer the clients stayed in the therapeutic community program, the less likely they were to use drugs and the more likely they were to be employed and to have committed no crimes. In a meta-analysis to determine the effectiveness of educational interventions on selected outcomes for diabetic patients, Brown (1992) found that the length of the educational intervention (measured in minutes) was associated with larger effect sizes for knowledge and skill performance. In the SHIP study, the number of classes attended by the women assigned to this experimental group had a positive effect on the rate of change in the ability for self-care, meaning that women who attended most of the classes showed the greatest improvement in their self-care over the one-year follow-up period (Sidani, 1994). Using the level of treatment as the independent variable predicting the outcomes, instead of the usual group dichotomy, increases the statistical power by an estimated amount of 10% (Cook & Poole, 1982). Despite its advantage, this approach for analyzing the effects of the intervention as delivered should be used cautiously since it may introduce bias in estimating treatment effects. The possible bias is associated with participants' self-selection into the levels of exposure to the treatment, resulting from variability on some client characteristics (Lipsey, 1990; Mark, 1983). The effects of the mediating variables on the expected outcomes can be examined using regression or path analysis. The processes underlying the effects of the intervention are represented in a causal model that specifies the links between the treatment variables measured by the type and intensity of the treatment received by each participant, the mediating variable(s), and the outcome variable(s). The links between the variables are represented in a causal chain showing that the outcome variables are regressed on the mediating variables and the mediating variables on the treatment variables. The regression or path coefficients are examined for significance to determine the magnitude of the hypothesized effects. It is expected that (a) the treatment exerts no effect on the outcome variables when the mediating variables are controlled, and (b) the coefficients of the path between the treatment and the mediating variables and between the mediating variables and outcome variables are statistically different from zero (Judd & Kenny, 1981, p. 606). The weaknesses of regression and path analysis relate to their limitations in estimating all the mediating processes simultaneously and in estimating the extent of measurement error. Structural equations modeling is an alternative approach for testing the mediational processes underlying an intervention effects. It has the advantages of assessing all hypothesized path coefficients simultaneously and of representing multiple indicators of mediating and outcome constructs if available, which reduces, or at least permits estimation of, measurement error. For a detailed presentation of structural equations models refer to Bentler (1992) and Hoyle (1995). The mediating processes can be tested (a) using the data gathered from all participants, with participants in the control group being assigned a value of zero on the treatment strength variable, which, in turn, is used to predict the mediating variables in the causal chain; or (b) in each group separately, comparing between the groups the estimated path coefficients linking the mediating to the outcome variables. Structural equations modeling permits the estimation of these parameters simultaneously in multiple groups and testing for the significance of any difference observed in the parameter estimates (Bentler, 1992; Judd & Kenny, 1981).

It is important to explain that the strategies and methods for maintaining and monitoring the integrity of the intervention implementation and for gathering process evaluation data, as described earlier, must be considered and specified before the actual intervention delivery. That is, they should be incorporated in the effectiveness study design and carried out properly if they are to be effective and useful in ensuring integrity and providing data about the treatment as delivered and the processes mediating the intervention effects. The intervention as delivered and the process data are then used in the analyses conducted to determine the intervention effectiveness in producing the desired outcomes.

The absence of an a priori plan makes difficult the identification and measurement of the intervention as delivered and the process variables and consequently the quantitative analysis of their effects. The qualitative approach for data collection and analysis can be used, however, to identify what actually happened during the intervention delivery, that is, what services or activities were offered for which purpose or to achieve which outcome, what problems were encountered during the implementation of the intervention, how these problems might have influenced the delivery of the intervention and the achievement of the outcomes, how clients perceived and responded to the intervention, what materials were used for delivering the intervention, and in what type of setting it was delivered. The qualitative data can be obtained from the interveners and the participants. The results can be used to provide a post hoc explanation of the observed intervention effects. For example, if the results of an effectiveness study indicated that the intervention did not produce the desired outcomes, then the findings of qualitative interviews may point to possible reason(s) explaining the lack of its effectiveness. Interveners may reveal that they were not able to deliver the intervention as specified in the protocol to all participants in the experimental group due to the frequent inadequate functioning of the equipment, for instance.

Advantages of Process Evaluation

Process evaluation provides data related to the characteristics of the clients who participated in or received the intervention, the features of the setting in which the treatment is delivered, the characteristics of the interveners, the nature of the interaction between interveners and participants, the reaction of participants to the intervention, the intervention component and the strength at which it was received, and the variables mediating the treatment effects. Examining the influence of these factors on outcomes increases our understanding of what really contributed to outcomes achievement. Such knowledge improves the validity of conclusions regarding intervention effectiveness and identifies factors required for a successful delivery of the treatment and successful outcomes achievement (Boruch & Gomez, 1977; Green & Lewis, 1986; Pauley & Cohen, 1984; Siderovski & Siderovski, 1992; Trochim, 1985). Judd and Kenny (1981) presented three advantages of process analysis. First, specifying and examining the mechanisms mediating the intervention effects increase our knowledge about the genesis of the outcome of interest. Analysis of the processes underlying the intervention effects allows not only examination of the treatment effects but also building and testing a theory of the general causal mechanisms responsible for producing the outcomes. Second, having a theoretical causal model for the outcome enhances the generalizability of the results of effectiveness research to other settings, populations, and treatments. In other words, a clear understanding of how the treatment effects are produced improves our ability to better predict whether the same effects will be produced in other contexts and under different conditions. Finally, knowledge of the intervention processes and the variables that have a direct impact on the outcomes of interest assists in designing more efficient interventions.

Summary

Process analysis, guided by the intervention theory, enhances our understanding of how the intervention works and which components of the intervention, at which intensity, result in which outcomes, for which client population, and under what conditions. Thus, process analysis assists in developing the clinical knowledge needed for providing high-quality care. It also improves the internal and external validity of effectiveness research. Conducting process analysis is not an easy task; it requires gathering an extensive amount of data and careful data management and analysis. But its advantages are worth the efforts.

Chapter 7

OUTCOMES-RELATED FACTORS

Clinicians, just like researchers, want to be confident that the observed changes in the clients' status are those expected as a result of the intervention and that they reflect true changes and not mere random fluctuations in the outcomes of interest. Obtaining such evidence depends on selecting the right outcomes variables, on selecting the right instruments that measure the intended outcomes accurately and with minimal error and that are sensitive to changes in the outcomes, and on selecting the right time for measuring the outcomes after the implementation of the intervention. These issues, if not addressed properly, reduce the likelihood of detecting real intervention effects when they are present and consequently threaten the validity of conclusions regarding the effectiveness of the intervention.

This chapter focuses on outcomes-related factors that influence the validity of conclusions in intervention effectiveness research. The characteristics of outcomes are introduced, as they may assist in the appropriate selection of outcomes. The issues of selecting outcomes variables and outcomes measures and the timing of outcomes measurement are discussed, and strategies for addressing or dealing with them are advanced. Finally, the influence of outcomes measurement on the validity of findings is illustrated with an example from the SHIP study.

Characteristics of Outcomes

Health-related outcomes are consequences or effects of interventions, manifested by changes in any dimensions of health or resolution of the presenting problem for which the intervention is given (Hegyvary, 1993; Lohr, 1988; Martin & Scheet, 1992). Changes in a health condition are represented by modifications in the level of the outcomes variable measured after the intervention delivery, compared against its level when measured before the intervention. Resolution of the presenting problem is reflected by its absence after the intervention. Thus, the effects of some interventions are manifested by changes in scores on the outcome variable, whereas the effects of other interventions, such as those designed to prevent complications, are manifested by absence or lack of occurrence or development of the particular complication or by maintaining the same level or score on the outcome variable. The outcomes expected of health or nursing interventions vary with the nature (i.e., the purpose, rationale, and type), the level of complexity, and the strength of the particular intervention being evaluated. For instance, the outcomes of a comprehensive cardiac rehabilitation program, with services offered over a 3-month period, close supervision of clients' activities, and monitoring of their health status, are numerous, tapping multiple domains of health. The changes in the clients' health status are expected to be maintained over one year after the provision of all the services. In contrast, an unstructured cardiac exercise program that provided minimal instructions about the type of exercises to be performed or about their frequency and duration is expected to produce small, nonsignificant changes in the clients' level of physical functioning that may not be sustained. The outcomes differ in their nature, in the time at which they are anticipated to occur and in the pattern of change over time, and in their specificity.

Nature of Outcomes

Different outcomes are of interest to health or nursing care professionals. They can be broadly categorized into (a) clinical end points related to the clients' response to health interventions, such as signs and symptoms, laboratory values, mortality, and complications; (b) functional status related to the maintenance or improvement of physical, mental, and social functioning; (c) perceptual outcomes related to the clients' general well-being and life satisfaction as well as the clients' satisfaction with the results of care, with the care received, and with the providers of care; and (d) financial outcomes related to use of resources and cost (Brooten & Naylor, 1995; Burrows-Hudson, 1995; Hegyvary, 1991; Lang & Marek, 1991; Mitchell, 1993; Russell & Buckwalter, 1991; Tarlov et al., 1989). This categorization of outcome is not meant to be exhaustive or prescriptive. In fact, a classification of patient outcomes that are sensitive to nursing interventions is being developed that may identify new categories of outcomes (Maas, Johnson, & Moorhead, 1996).

Within these categories, outcomes can be objective or subjective. Objective outcomes include variables such as laboratory values and cost. Data on these variables can be obtained from sources other than the client. Subjective outcomes include variables such as sense of well-being and functional status. Data from these outcomes are perceptual, requiring the client's personal judgment or expression of thoughts, feelings, or attitudes.

The changes observed after the implementation of the treatment can represent intended or unintended outcomes of the intervention. The intended outcomes are the desired effects that the intervention strives to achieve. They reflect the purpose(s) for which the intervention was delivered and therefore are used as criteria to assess its effectiveness. Unintended outcomes are the changes that occur as a result of the intervention but were not anticipated or hypothesized by the researcher or the clinician (Chen, 1990). For example, in a pilot study conducted to evaluate the effectiveness of listening to music, the intended outcome was a reduction in the level of anxiety experienced by clients with chronic obstructive pulmonary disease. Some clients reported going to sleep after listening to music, which was an unanticipated, though beneficial, outcome (Sidani, 1991).

The identification of the particular outcomes expected of an intervention is guided by the intervention theory underlying its effects. The theory specifies the problem requiring the intervention, the purpose for which the intervention is given, and its anticipated effects. The intended outcomes are derived from these elements of the intervention theory. Unintended outcomes can be identified from findings of previous studies that evaluated the intervention effects, from research, or from clinicians' "best guesses" or working hypotheses. Qualitative methods are the most appropriate for identifying unintended intervention outcomes, since qualitative methods encourage putting aside any preconceived notion or a priori knowledge about the intervention effects, which facilitates exploration of how the clients have been affected by the intervention.

Timing and Pattern of Change

Outcomes achievement is anticipated to occur at different points in time after treatment delivery. Changes in some outcomes are expected to occur immediately after the implementation of the intervention, whereas changes in others take some time to appear. The onset of changes in the outcomes varies. Some changes may have an abrupt onset, and others exhibit a more gradual onset. In addition, the extent to which changes in the outcomes are maintained over a specified period of time differs. Some changes may be of short duration, whereas others may be sustained over long periods of time. Taken together, time, onset, and maintenance of changes are aspects of outcomes achievement that can be combined to reflect the pattern of change in the outcomes variables. The pattern of change in outcomes is not uniform. Some outcomes may demonstrate an abrupt onset of changes occurring immediately after the intervention is given and be maintained for a one-year period. Other outcomes may show gradual onset that peaks at some point in time after the intervention (Lipsey, 1993). Figure 7.1 provides hypothetical examples of patterns of change in outcomes.

The pattern of change in outcomes is related to the purpose of the intervention, its components or activities, and its strength. For example, outcomes of interventions with a behavioral component that aim at enhancing the clients' stress management skills may show a pattern of delayed onset of the changes that peak few months after the intervention delivery and are sustained for one year. This intervention component requires the clients to learn the behavioral skills through intensive training; once a behavior is learned, however, it becomes part of the repertoire of skills that the client has.

The pattern of change in outcomes is determined by the intervention theory. Knowledge of the critical inputs (component, mode of delivery, and dosage) and of the chain of processes linking the intervention to outcomes are necessary for delineating the outcomes' pattern of change. To illustrate this point, interventions that consist of one component that does not demand sophisticated skills to carry it out by the interveners or participants,

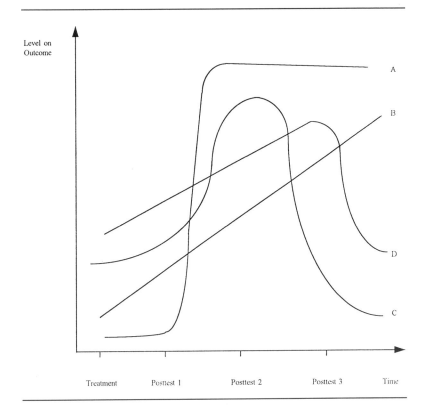

Figure 7.1: Patterns of Change in Outcomes

that are strong, and that have a short causal chain linking them to the outcomes are expected to demonstrate a pattern similar to Pattern A in Figure 7.1. When the intervention theory is lacking, the pattern of change in the outcomes can be empirically derived from previous or current effectiveness studies.

The pattern of outcomes change hypothesized by the intervention theory can be compared to the pattern of change observed empirically in the effectiveness study. For instance, knowledge related to cancer and its treatment and the ability for self-care were two outcomes of the SHIP interventions. The hypothesized pattern of change in knowledge was similar to Pattern A in Figure 7.1, whereas the one for self-care resembled Pattern B. The hypothesized and observed patterns of change in these outcomes were congruent. The level of knowledge gained increased immediately after the implementation of the intervention and was subsequently maintained during the follow-up period in most participants. The reported level of self-care ability showed a gradual increase over time, with the highest level achieved one year posttest (Sidani, 1994).

Specificity

Variables that reflect outcomes of health or nursing interventions are numerous. These outcome variables and the instruments measuring them vary in their specificity in relation to the particular intervention being evaluated. They can be either generic or specific. Generic outcome measures include (a) a global indicator of the concept of interest, such as a single question about the clients' perception of their overall health status; (b) a multiple-item measure reflective of all domains of the concept of interest and inquiring about the clients' response in general, not in relation to the specific condition they are in (e.g., a general measure of functional status, such as the Sickness Impact Profile, SIP); and (c) general indicators of quality of care that are considered as criteria for evaluating the effectiveness of health care, such as mortality rate or satisfaction with care. Specific outcomes measures focus on aspects of the concept that are of primary interest to the situation being assessed. The specific aspects measured are only those expected of the intervention, such as assessing physical functioning in relation to a cardiac exercise program. The instruments used may be adapted to the specific presenting problem for which the intervention is given, to the specific client population receiving the treatment, or to the specific disease that participants have. For example, the questions pertinent to physical functioning in the SIP can be tailored to elicit responses with reference to the cardiac condition experienced by participants in the cardiac exercise program (Guyatt, Feeny, & Patrick, 1993).

In summary, outcomes of interest in effectiveness research represent various dimensions of health, at different levels of specificity in relation to the intervention, to the presenting problem, or to the client population involved in the situation being evaluated, and are expected to show different patterns of change over time. The variability in the characteristics of outcomes affects the selection of outcomes variables, outcomes measures, and the timing for measuring the outcomes postintervention.

Selection of Outcomes Variables

Outcomes have the advantage of being comprehensive in that they reflect all their antecedents. Outcomes are affected not only by the intervention that was delivered to participants but also by a host of factors related to the preexisting personal characteristics of the clients, to the humanistic or interpersonal characteristics of the intervener, and to the setting in which the care is provided (Donabedian, 1988; Peters, 1988). Clinical reality shows that outcomes may vary regardless of the care given; for example, the clients' health status may improve or deteriorate irrespective of the treatments delivered (Bond & Thomas, 1991; Hegyvary, 1991; Taylor, 1974). The advantage of comprehensiveness in reflecting all antecedents presents a challenge in selecting outcome variables in effectiveness research.

The conventional, outcomes-focused approach to effectiveness research met this challenge by selecting multiple, generic outcomes to reflect the intervention effects. Examples of such generic outcomes are mortality, morbidity, number of patient complications developed during a stay in a health care facility, length of stay in the facility, number of readmissions (Closs & Tierney, 1993; Raskin & Maklan, 1991; Zinn, Aaronson, & Rosko, 1993), functional status, mental status, stress level, satisfaction with care, patients' knowledge of self-management, well-being, quality of life, and return to work (Brooten & Naylor, 1995; Closs & Tierney, 1993; French, 1995). These generic outcomes are measured with global outcomes measures inquiring about the clients' responses in general, irrespective of the specific health domain that is expected to be affected by the nature (i.e., purpose, mechanisms, activities or components) of the intervention being evaluated.

Selecting multiple global outcomes when evaluating particular interventions may be advantageous. These global outcomes are considered standard criteria for assessing the impact of intervention of programs of health care. They represent the direct and indirect benefits for the individual and society. Thus, they are of interest to health care payers and policymakers (French, 1995; Raskin & Maklan, 1991). Furthermore, these outcomes criteria permit comparisons of different interventions or programs addressing the same presenting problem. These comparisons are required for clinical and administrative decision making, such as selecting the intervention that is most effective and efficient in producing a desired outcome.

Last, generic outcomes cover various domains of health, some of which may not be anticipated to be affected by a particular intervention. Thus, including generic outcomes may facilitate the detection of unintended outcomes. Nonetheless, generic outcomes are often influenced by factors other than the intervention being evaluated. For example, return to work is contingent on the clients' employment status and the employer's decision, not only on the intervention success. Furthermore, generic outcomes are, for the most part, far removed from the nature of the intervention; that is, they do not focus on the area of interest, making it difficult if not impossible to link them conceptually to the intervention. Even if directly linked and specifically addressed by the intervention, generic outcomes are less likely to undergo clinically important changes as a result of the intervention (Guyatt et al., 1993; Stewart & Archbold, 1992). For example, changes in life satisfaction may not be expected to occur as a result of an educational intervention concerned with providing knowledge about a disease and its treatment only. It may result from, say, changes in social status as well. In addition, examining the effects of the intervention on multiple generic outcomes runs the risk of committing Type I error. Conducting multiple statistical tests to determine the effect of the intervention on each generic outcomes variable increases the probability that one of the obtained effect sizes will be significant by chance alone, leading to erroneous conclusions about the intervention effectiveness. A stringent level of significance may be preset to reduce Type I error associated with repeated testing. Unfortunately, a stringent level of significance decreases the power of detecting real effects if present, with the potential for Type II error (Cohen, 1982).

Although generic outcomes are useful to assess the quality of health care at a macro level of analysis, such as when examining the impact of a new nursing care delivery system, they may be inappropriate for evaluating the effects of a particular intervention on the health of individual clients (Jones, 1993). What is needed at this relatively micro level of analysis are outcomes that represent the clients' response to the specific treatment given to resolve specific presenting problems (Mitchell, 1993). Thus, specific rather than generic outcomes variables have to be selected. Specific outcomes are more likely to be responsive to the particular intervention being evaluated and sensitive to the condition of the particular clients who receive it. They are linked to the intervention and are specific to the presenting problem and to the client population involved in the effectiveness study.

Therefore, including specific outcomes increases the likelihood that significant intervention effects will be detected, if present, and are responsive to clinically relevant changes that are of interest to both clinicians and patients. Furthermore, including only relevant outcomes reduces the chances of committing Type I error. Despite its advantages, focusing on specific outcomes has two disadvantages. The first is limited ability to compare different interventions addressing the same presenting problem in different client populations or in different conditions, since different outcome criteria, adapted to a particular client population or condition, may be used when evaluating each intervention (Guyatt et al., 1993). The second is inability to detect unintended outcomes of the intervention, since the focus is on the expected ones only. Knowledge of the unintended effects of an intervention is important for clinical decision making.

   In the alternative, theory-driven approach to effectiveness research, the selection of specific outcomes is guided by the intervention theory. The outcomes are derived from the nature of the presenting problem, the purpose of the intervention and its components, the processes mediating its effects, and the expected outcomes as specified in the theory. That is, the intervention theory defines the problem for which the intervention is given, specifies what activities need to be done to deal with the presenting problem and what consequences (i.e., changes in particular domains of health) are expected as a result of the activities performed, and explains how the activities lead to the expected consequences. These elements of the intervention theory point to the outcomes expected of the intervention. Furthermore, the theory of complex, multicomponent interventions or programs specifies which particular outcome(s) is (are) influenced by which specific intervention component(s). Rosen and Proctor (1978) considered the key mediating variables, identified in the intervention theory, as intermediate outcomes and the intended effects as ultimate outcomes. Intermediate outcomes are those changes that result from the intervention that are presumed to contribute to or create a facilitative climate for the attainment of the ultimate outcomes. They are the direct products of the intervention activities. Ultimate outcomes represent the set of treatment objectives. They constitute the reasons for which the treatment is given (Rosen & Proctor, 1978). In the example of the stress management educational intervention, knowledge of stress management techniques is considered the intermediate outcome, since learning how to apply the techniques facilitates their use. Daily use of the techniques can be viewed as a second intermediate outcome that may lead to improved sense of psychological well-being. Well-being represents the ultimate outcome of this intervention. The relationship among the intervention and the different outcomes variables can be represented in a causal diagram (as discussed in Chapter 3) and empirically tested (Lipsey, 1993).

In the example of the uncertainty management intervention (UMI) of the SHIP study, the uncertainty theory predicted that (a) the cognitive component of the UMI increases knowledge related to cancer and its treatment and strengthens the women's cognitive structure (intermediate outcomes), which, in turn, promote their appraisal of the uncertainty as a challenge for growth rather than as danger (a challenge appraisal reduces the level of uncertainty and consequently improves psychological adjustment—ultimate outcomes); (b) the psychological component of the UMI reduces emotional distress; and (c) the behavioral component enhances the women's uncertainty management skills these two intermediate outcomes of the psychological and behavioral components reduce the level of uncertainty experienced by the women, which improves their psychological adjustment to cancer.

The theoretical approach to selecting outcomes increases the likelihood that the outcomes identified are relevant, specific, and sensitive to the intended effects of the intervention or its components, enhancing the construct validity of the effectiveness study conclusions. Furthermore, the intervention theory may point to possible unintended effects, as discussed earlier in this chapter. A priori identification of unintended outcomes permits their measurement; consequently, their association with the intervention can be examined. Results of such analyses provide for a comprehensive understanding and empirical support of how the intervention works to produce which outcomes, leading to further support of the intervention theory or to its refinement.

Selection of Outcomes Measures

Once the outcomes, intermediate (i.e., key mediating variables) and ultimate (i.e., intended effects), expected of the intervention are identified, they have to be operationalized and measured in an effectiveness study to provide the data needed to test the intervention effectiveness in producing the desired outcomes. Selecting instruments to measure the identified outcome variables is another outcomes-related factor with the potential to threaten the validity of conclusions regarding the intervention effectiveness. The instruments to be selected should (a) represent accurately the intended effects of the intervention, (b) be responsive to clinically relevant changes, and (c) be maximally responsive to the intervention effects and minimally responsive to other factors with a direct influence on the expected changes. Instruments that do not validly measure the intended intervention outcomes and that do not capture true changes in the outcomes may not be responsive to the intervention effects: They cannot detect significant or real changes in the intended outcomes, potentially leading to erroneous conclusions.

Instruments that are responsive to the intended intervention effects must have the following properties: construct validity; validity for detecting change; sensitivity to change, or responsiveness; and reliability.

Construct Validity

A valid instrument measures what it purports to measure—that is, it measures the right phenomenon or attribute. In effectiveness research, the instrument selected must have validity for measuring the outcomes variable the intervention is expected to change. Therefore, the content of the instrument used to operationalize the outcomes variable must be congruent with its conceptual definition. The intervention theory presents conceptual definitions of the outcomes variables. Clear and specific conceptual definitions lead to increased specificity of outcomes measurement and consequently increased responsiveness of the outcomes measure (Trochim, 1985). Congruence between the theoretical and operational definitions of outcomes is best examined by assessing the construct validity of the instrument. An instrument with established construct validity represents all domains of the variable, does not capture irrelevancies in the responses associated with the method of data collection, and is minimally responsive to other distinct constructs that may influence the subjects' responses (Messick, 1995). Outcomes measures should be also valid in relation to the population studied. They should represent all the domains of the construct of interest in a way that is applicable and relevant to the specific client population (Hegyvary, 1993; Russell & Buckwalter, 1991). For instance, self-care activities that could be performed by a young adult or life events a young adult encounters differ from those expected for an older adult.

Selecting valid outcomes measures starts by defining the changes expected to result from the treatment. Once defined, available instrument(s) measuring the domains(s) of the outcome concept are identified and evaluated for construct validity. Evaluating construct validity involves judging the degree of fit between the content areas covered by the measure with those identified in the definition of the expected changes and reviewing previous research findings to determine whether the measures have demonstrated validity (Lipsey, 1990). When the available empirical evidence of validity is insufficient or inconclusive, the investigator can (a) conduct a pilot study to assess the validity of the selected measures, using either correlational analyses or criterion group contrast; (b) measure the outcomes variable in the effectiveness study using multiple indicators of the same and of distinct but related concepts, using different methods or sources of data collection (this approach, which is similar to the multitrait-multimethod approach to construct validation enhances validity by reducing method bias) (Sechrest et al., 1983); or (c) develop relevant measures. Some scholars advocate developing instruments that validly measure the specific attributes that are likely to undergo changes as a result of the intervention and that are responsive only to the changes brought about by the treatment (Guyatt, Deyo, Charlson, Levine, & Mitchell, 1989; Stewart & Archbold, 1992). These types of measures have been broadly called *edumetric measures* (Carver, 1974). Edumetric measures are those measures "developed by sampling some defined content domain which represents the new responses subjects are expected to acquire as a result of the treatment" (Lipsey, 1990, p. 103). They draw upon salient aspects of the attribute or concept that are likely to undergo clinically important changes following the implementation of the intervention. Criterion-referenced tests (Waltz, Strickland, & Lenz, 1991), such as tests used to assess the knowledge of a disease and its treatment gained by participants who attended an educational session addressing these specific topics, are examples of edumetric measures. Participants are expected to score low on this measure at pretest, since they do not possess the knowledge they are being tested on, and to score high at posttest, reflecting their knowledge gain and indicating the effectiveness of the intervention.

For instance, in the SHIP study, cancer-related knowledge was identified as an outcome expected of the self-help and uncertainty management interventions. Cancer-related knowledge was measured by a 24-item scale developed by the investigators (Braden et al., 1989) to assess the women's understanding of the disease pathophysiology, symptomatology, treatment, prognosis, and self-care activities. The items were derived from the content discussed in the self-help classes and the phone contacts. The items consisted of statements about the meaning of words commonly used in written materials about breast cancer, breast anatomy, characteristics of cancer cells, treatment protocols, common side effects of treatment, and activities that are used to care for self. Thus, this cancer-related knowledge scale sampled information given to women who received the interventions and were expected to change following the intervention (i.e., women were expected to gain more information related to cancer, its treatment, and self-care after the intervention delivery). The scores on the knowledge scale were relatively low and did not differ significantly across the three groups of participants at pretest; the mean scores were 14.4 for the self-help classes, 14.8 for the uncertainty management intervention (UMI), and 12.8 for the control group. The scores changed significantly at posttest for the self-help classes (mean score posttest = 19.3) and the UMI (mean score posttest = 16.2), but not for the control group (mean score = 14.6). This pattern of change in knowledge scores, which is typical for edumetric measures, indicates that the knowledge scale validly captured the women's expected response to the intervention.

Goal-attainment scales are another example of edumetric measures. They can be used when the outcomes variable, such as symptoms, is both the indicator for and the outcome of treatment or when the intervention and expected outcomes are tailored to the individual needs of clients (Lang & Marek, 1990; Malec, Smigielski, & DePompolo, 1991; Stewart & Archbold, 1992). Goal-attainment scaling techniques consist of developing outcomes that are linked to the presenting problem for which the treatment is given and assessing the clients' improvement toward achieving these outcomes. Participants may be asked to indicate whether their condition is "better," "worse," or "the same" postintervention to determine where they stand on each problem-outcome link. The rating can be also done by the clinicians or interveners (Deyo & Inui, 1984; Inzer & Aspinal, 1981).

Validity for Detecting Change

In addition to construct validity, which is essential for detecting the changes that are specific and sensitive to the intervention, outcomes measures must be valid for detecting true intraindividual changes in the expected outcomes—that is, the "measures show an observable difference when there is, in fact, a change on the characteristic measured that is of sufficient magnitude to be interesting in the context of application" (Lipsey, 1990, p. 100). In other words, observed changes in the participants' responses or scores on the outcomes measures should reflect expected changes in the characteristic being measured and not random fluctuations attributable to situational variability (Guyatt, Kirshner, & Jaeschke, 1992).

Assessing a measure's validity for detecting true changes in the outcomes is not an easy task since few methods are available to carry such analyses. The strategies proposed for examining validity for detecting change rely on judging the congruence between the expected, hypothesized changes and the empirical, observed ones. Carver (1974) suggested comparing the degree of actual gain to the degree of expected gain in order to estimate what he called *edumetric validity*. The hypothesized or expected gain is derived from the intervention theory or from previous findings and is proportional to the strength of the intervention. Deyo and Inui (1984), Kirshner and Guyatt (1985), and Deyo and Centor (1986) proposed other methods for assessing the ability of outcomes measures to detect significant changes. The simplest method consists of examining changes in the outcomes measure scores following an intervention of *known efficacy*. The amount of change observed between pretest and posttest would indicate the scale's ability to detect change. This method is similar to the one proposed by Carver (1974), since the changes expected as a result of an intervention with known efficacy are known a priori and can be compared to the ones obtained. The second strategy consists of obtaining change scores on the outcomes measure and scores on a criterion measure indexing change. The criterion measure could be other relevant data indicating improvement in the participants' status, such as the scores on a goal-attainment scale indicating the level of improvement in status. The data can be analyzed by correlating the outcomes change scores with the criterion measure scores or by conducting sensitivity and specificity analyses.

Sensitivity and specificity analyses provide information about the accuracy of the outcomes measure in detecting true change. For example, when evaluating the effectiveness of a rehabilitation program for patients with lung diseases, the SIP can be used as a measure of functional status; improved functional status is identified as an outcome of this program. To determine the validity of the SIP in detecting true changes in functional status, patients are asked to complete the SIP and to indicate how much they improved in performing activities of daily living at the end of the program period. The data can be analyzed in two ways. First, the change scores on the SIP are correlated with the scores on the improvement rating scale. Positive strong correlations indicate that the SIP is valid in detecting changes. Second, sensitivity and specificity analysis is conducted. In this analysis, a cutoff score for the SIP is identified from the scale's normative values (if available) or from the investigators or clinicians' expert judgment of which score indicates clinically relevant change. Participants are then classified into those who improved and those who deteriorated, based on their SIP and self-rating scores. High sensitivity and specificity indexes indicate that the SIP score is accurate in differentiating between those who did and did not improve.

Despite their advantages, sensitivity and specificity analyses have some limitations. First, it is sometimes difficult to find a meaningful cutoff score that is able to distinguish between different levels of change in the outcome, especially when the outcome is perceptual, such as quality of life. Second, the validity of the findings depends on the validity of the criterion index of change used. For example, the participants' self-rating of improvement may be biased. Last, and most important, the sensitivity and specificity analyses require dichotomization of the outcomes scores and of the criterion index of change. Such dichotomization results in loss of information and reduces the ability to detect true but small changes. For instance, those who reported being the same are excluded from the analyses or lumped with those who improved or did not improve. Finally, a measure can lack validity for change (a) if it is scaled in units that are too gross to detect the expected change (e.g., using a categorical scaling method to measure a continuous variable is inadequate and is less sensitive to change than a graduated scale, since the former only records change between categories, not within them); and (b) if it has floor or ceiling effect so that all participants select the same response or demonstrate high or low scores at different points in time, thus limiting downward or upward change in the responses over time (Lipsey, 1990).

Sensitivity to Change, or Responsiveness

For the outcomes measures to be responsive to the intervention effects, they should be also sensitive to change. Sensitivity to change, or responsiveness, means ability to capture interindividual differences in the outcomes: Measures should be sensitive to differences in the outcomes between participants who received and those who did not receive the intervention (Stewart & Archbold, 1993). Differences in the outcome variable observed after the implementation of the intervention can be due to true interindividual differences between the participants or to the intervention effects, however. True interindividual differences are associated with some extraneous factors, such as personal or health characteristics of clients. These true interindividual differences that are not associated with the intervention effects contribute to the undesirable within-experimental group variance, which obscures or confounds the intervention effects. Therefore, the instruments needed in effectiveness research should be able to capture the responses participants are expected to acquire as a result of the intervention, and not the interindividual differences related to extraneous factors. That is, they should be more sensitive to the changes induced by the treatment and less sensitive to preexisting individual differences on the characteristic being measured (Lipsey, 1990). Consequently, such measures should show low interindividual variability at both pretest and posttest. Low variability at pretest indicates minimal individual differences in the outcomes variable (i.e., the participants are equivalent on this variable). At posttest, low variability in the outcomes measure is desirable in the experimental group. Low variability in the experimental group indicates uniformity in the participants' response to the treatment (i.e., the treatment should add a constant value on the outcome variable score if it is equally effective for all subjects). When participants respond in the same way, within-experimental group variance in the outcome is reduced, increasing statistical power for detecting significant intervention effects. Low variability is manifested by low reliability coefficients computed using the scores of participants in the experimental group (Nicewander & Price, 1983). Variability in the outcomes measure scores is expected, however, when examining the distribution of scores obtained from participants in the experimental and control groups. This variability reflects the differences in the outcomes scores between participants in the experimental and control groups and results in high reliability coefficients computed using the total sample scores (Bejar, 1980; Stucliffe, 1980). To illustrate this point, the alpha coefficient for one of the major outcomes variables in the SHIP study was computed for the total sample, one experimental group, and the control group, over time. For the total sample, the alpha coefficient was .84 at pretest; .84 immediately posttest; and 3 months after posttest,

.87. For the treatment group, the alpha coefficient was .83, .78, and .84, respectively. For the control group, the alpha coefficient was .85, .85, and .86 at the three points in time. The small drop in the alpha coefficient immediately posttest in the treatment group suggests low interindividual differences in the outcomes measure, reflecting some homogeneity of responses to treatment. In contrast, no changes in the alpha coefficient were observed over time in the control group, as expected. The relatively high alpha coefficients at posttest in the total sample indicate increased differences between the groups on this outcome, suggesting that the intervention was effective. But the large coefficient observed at pretest implies the presence of preexisting interindividual differences, which weakens the confidence in claiming that this outcomes measure was maximally responsive to the treatment effects and minimally responsive to true individual differences at posttest. Therefore, measures that are designed to capture true interindividual differences are not necessarily responsive to treatment effects. Edumetric measures are considered more sensitive to changes induced by the intervention and less sensitive to preexisting individual differences, because they measure the specific characteristics that participants are expected to lack before the intervention and to gain after it. Thus, they capture the differences in the outcomes attributed to the intervention only.

Reliability

A measure must be reliable to be sensitive to interindividual differences, to detect true changes, and to reflect the outcomes accurately. A reliable instrument measures the outcomes variable with consistency and minimal error. Error represents fluctuations in the measure scores that are unrelated to the characteristic being measured. These fluctuations could be random or systematic. Random error of measurement is due to chance factors related to the properties of the measure or its application, such as the type of items included in a self-report measure, the clarity of the content covered, the clarity and specificity of the instructions provided, typing errors, the manner in which the responses are coded and scored, subjects' guessing, and poorly functioning physical or mechanical instruments. Random error can also be procedural, associated with inconsistent application of the measure across participants. Sources of procedural error include (a) the subjects' condition at the time of administering the measure, such as their attention span, level of anxiety, motivation, or fatigue; and (b) the conditions under which the measurement is done, such as the location of measurement, the heat or lighting in the room, the length of the measurement procedure (i.e., an increase in the length of time taken to respond to numerous scales potentially leads to respondents' fatigue), and the time at which the measure was administered. Systematic error results in bias and is related to such factors as the subjects' general ability to comprehend instructions, test-taking skills, reading ability, acquiescence, or social desirability (Lipsey, 1990; Waltz et al., 1991).

Error of measurement, whether random or systematic, increases the variability in the distribution of scores on the outcomes measure for subjects in the experimental and control groups. This variability is undesirable, however, since it is associated with neither the characteristic being measured nor the treatment effects. Thus, it contributes to the within-group variance, increasing the error variance in tests of statistical significance. The net result is decreased power for detecting significant intervention effects. Methods for reducing error of measurement vary with its source. In general, they involve maintaining consistency in administering the measure to all participants; carefully reviewing the measure for clarity, format, and content before administering it; developing and following systematic coding and scoring procedure; measuring social desirability and estimating its effects on the subjects' responses; using multiple indicators of the same concept (either multiple items or multiple measures); and aggregating or averaging scores to reflect the concept of interest. By aggregating multiple indicators, the error or bias inherent in each is counterbalanced and therefore reduced. Efforts to reduce the undesirable variability in outcomes measures may not be always successful. A large error variance may be present, leading to nonsignificant findings. In such situations, it is worth examining the reliability of the outcomes measures used in the effectiveness study and determining whether the error variance is due to measurement error or to preexisting true interindividual differences (subject heterogeneity) on the outcomes measure.

Assessing the reliability of the outcome measures provides information about the extent of measurement error still present despite the application of strategies to minimize it. Assessing the reliability of measures involves determining their internal consistency, test-retest stability, or interrater reliability. In effectiveness research, it may be inappropriate to expect and use outcomes measures with high test-retest reliability. High test-retest reliability indicates that the measure is capable of reproducing the same scores for the same individuals over time. Such a measure may not be able to capture changes, but sensitivity to change is a property required of outcomes measures (Kirshner & Guyatt, 1985). The internal consistency and interrater reliability of outcomes measures need to be evaluated. Methods for assessing internal consistency include the split-half, the KR-20, the Cronbach's alpha coefficients, and factor analysis (Zeller & Carmines, 1980). Results of these analyses indicate which, if any, items contribute to error and should be eliminated from the scale total scores to reduce measurement error. Interrater reliability is assessed by computing the percent of agreement among the raters (Kappa coefficient) or the correlation between the ratings of the raters (Waltz et al., 1991).

Ways to differentiate the two sources of error (i.e., measurement error and interindividual differences) are based on partitioning the error variance into two components: the measurement component and the subject heterogeneity component. The contribution of each of these variance components to the total observed variance in a measure is examined, thus allowing one to identify the extent to which the components introduce error (Lipsey, 1990). Generalizability theory is an approach used to determine the influence of multiple sources of variance in measurement, such as the items, the persons, the measure or method, and the occasion of measurement. This approach consists of partitioning the total variance in the outcomes measure scores into variance components associated with the sources of measurement variance and determining the extent to which each source contributes to measurement error. A detailed discussion of generalizability theory is beyond the scope of this book (refer to Cronbach, Gleser, Nanda, & Rajaratnam, 1972; Shavelson & Webb, 1991; Shavelson, Webb, & Rowley, 1989).

In summary, outcomes measures should be valid in reflecting the characteristic that is expected to change as a result of the intervention, valid in detecting true changes, reliable, and responsive to the intervention effects and not to preexisting individual differences in the outcomes. Some scholars have argued that outcomes measures should not be discriminative, that is, able to distinguish between individuals with different levels on the outcomes; rather, they should be evaluative, that is, able to capture within-individual change in the level of outcomes. They also emphasize that a reliable measure (i.e., characterized by high discriminative ability) is not necessarily responsive to intraindividual change (Kirshner & Guyatt, 1985). The counterargument is that a responsive measure should be able to distinguish variations in the level of the characteristic in order to detect changes. An evaluative measure that is not able to discriminate differences in levels is of limited use. The differences in outcomes level should be validly attributed to the intervention effects and not to preexisting individual variations, however, which is a matter of conceptual attribution of the variance or interpreting the findings correctly, and not a matter of the inherent property of the measures (Williams & Naylor, 1992).

Timing for Outcomes Measurement

The timing for measuring the selected outcomes is another factor that may influence the validity of conclusions in effectiveness research. Timing refers to the point in time at which the outcomes are measured. In the conventional approach to effectiveness research, outcomes are measured prior to implementation of the intervention and at the conclusion of the treatment. Pretest measures are used to examine initial equivalence and as reference in determining if any change in outcomes took place at posttest, as well as the amount of that change when present. Measuring outcomes after the treatment is essential for detecting the expected intervention effects. Measuring the outcomes only once after the intervention delivery assumes that the treatment effects have an abrupt onset and peak immediately after treatment implementation. The expected changes in different outcomes variables might appear at different points in time after treatment delivery, however, with some changes most pronounced immediately after intervention and others at some later time. The pattern of change in the outcomes must be prespecified, based on the propositions of the intervention theory (as detailed earlier) to identify the points in time at which the outcomes should be assessed. In the absence of these prespecifications of patterns of change, "it is quite possible that even with careful research, an investigator will fail to detect important treatment effects simply by looking in the wrong place at the wrong time" (Lipsey, 1993, p. 20). The hypothesized patterns of change in outcomes guide the researcher in selecting the appropriate time for outcomes measurement, the number of times and the time interval between occasions of the measurement, and the length of period for follow-up posttreatment. Finally, repeated outcomes measurement facilitates the detection of the true pattern of change over time as discussed in Chapter 4.

Illustrative Example

The influence of outcomes measures on the validity of conclusions regarding intervention effectiveness is illustrated with an example from the SHIP study. The theoretical framework that guided the development of the self-help classes proposed that the class activities lead to changes in symptom pattern experienced by women with breast cancer receiving adjuvant therapy. The class activities included problem-solving activities that focused on assisting the women to identify physical and emotional problems or symptoms they may experience and to learn about their possible causes and about methods for managing them. Changes in symptom pattern were defined as reduction in the number, frequency, and severity of symptoms, as reported by the women. It was hypothesized that the changes in symptom pattern are most pronounced 3 months after implementation of the intervention, since the women need some time to learn and apply the problem-solving abilities. The Symptom Transition Scale (STS) was selected to measure symptom pattern. The STS is a 12-item, self-report measure assessing the degree to which symptoms are perceived to be in a state of change or transition. Five of the STS items are positively stated, indicating a decrease in the number, severity, duration, visibility, and intrusiveness of the symptoms experienced; seven items are negatively stated, indicating an increase in the type, visibility, intrusiveness, duration, number, and novelty of the symptoms experienced. The aspects of symptom pattern covered by the STS were congruent with the definition of this outcome as specified by the intervention theoretical framework. Thus, the STS was considered valid in capturing the intervention outcome of symptom pattern.

The scale has a five-point, Likert-type response format, ranging from *strongly disagree* to *strongly agree*. The scoring technique used is summated rating after necessary reverse-coding of the negatively stated items is done. Higher scale scores indicate improvement in symptom pattern (i.e., reduction in the symptom number and intrusiveness). The STS was reported as meeting the validity and reliability criteria for a newly developed scale. Symptom pattern was measured at three points in time: pretest (T1), immediately posttest (T2), and 3 months later (T3). The reliability of the STS was examined to determine the extent of, and to take necessary measures to minimize, measurement error prior to conducting analyses of the intervention effectiveness in producing the desired changes in symptom pattern. The internal consistency reliability of the STS was assessed using Cronbach's alpha coefficient. The STS alpha coefficient, based on pretest data obtained from 282 women who participated in the study, was .64. This value of the alpha coefficient is low and may imply potential measurement error.

The effect of this measurement error on the validity of conclusions was demonstrated by non-statistically significant changes in the symptom pattern scores across the three points of measurement and between the experimental and control groups. These findings implied that the intervention was not effective in producing the expected changes in symptom pattern. Further reliability and validity analyses (Braden, Sidani, Ferketich, & Verran, 1993) indicated that the STS items measure two distinct aspects of symptom pattern. One aspect measured symptom extension (i.e., the symptoms were perceived as "getting worse," measured by the negatively stated items), and the other measured symptom retrenchment (i.e., the symptoms were perceived as improving, measured by the positively stated items). As a result, two distinct subscales of the STS were formed, representing the two aspects of symptom pattern. The Cronbach's alpha for the subscales were .92 and .90, respectively. The repeated-measure ANOVA was conducted on each subscale. Results indicated a significant time main effect for the symptom extension subscale in which the most prominent changes occurred at T3 as hypothesized, indicating increased sensitivity of the scale to change in the level of symptom extension.

This example illustrates the importance of not only selecting appropriate outcomes measures but also assessing and maintaining their reliability and validity in effectiveness research. Measures with questionable reliability and validity are not sensitive to changes in the outcomes and therefore threaten the validity of conclusions regarding the effectiveness of the intervention being evaluated.

Summary

In conclusion, measuring the right outcomes variable, with the right instrument, and at the right time is necessary for determining the effectiveness of the intervention in producing the expected effects. The right outcomes variable represents the anticipated treatment effect. The right outcomes measure reflects the outcomes of interest accurately, with minimal error, and is able to detect the changes expected as a result of the intervention. The right time is the point in time at which the changes are expected to occur. The selection of the appropriate outcomes variable, outcomes measure, and timing for outcomes measurement is informed by the intervention theory. The theory identifies and defines the outcomes; describes their relationships with the intervention; and specifies the nature, extent, and pattern of changes in the outcomes. These specifications form the basis for selecting the measures and for interpreting the findings.

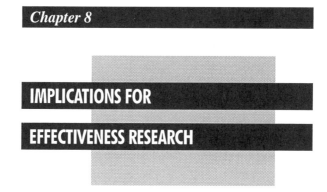

Chapter 8

IMPLICATIONS FOR
EFFECTIVENESS RESEARCH

The point made throughout this book is that providing high-quality care rests on the availability of a sound knowledge base of the problem(s) with which clients present and that require management and of the interventions that are effective in managing the presenting problem and producing desired outcomes. To be useful in guiding clinicians' practice and decision making, this knowledge base has to answer the clinically relevant questions of which intervention is effective, at what optimal dosage, with which clients, under what conditions, in producing which outcomes. Valid answers to these questions are developed from an interplay between theory and research. Theories explain the nature and etiology of the presenting problem; the nature of the intervention in terms of its components, dosage, and mode of delivery; the mechanisms through which the intervention produces its desired effects; and the conditions necessary for the proper implementation of the intervention and the intervention to achieve its intended outcomes. Theories remain an abstract conceptualization or representation of the world phenomena, reflecting the best guess of their developers until they are tested empirically. Research is the medium through which theories are tested. Research provides the empirical evidence that does or does not corroborate the propositions of theories or leads to their refinement.

Advantages of Theory-Driven Evaluation

The linkage between theory and research is exemplified by the theory-driven approach to effectiveness research, discussed in the previous chapters. The advantages of using the theory-driven approach are numerous. The theory guides the design, development, and delivery of the intervention. It guides the design of an effectiveness study and it informs the selection of participants, variables, and points in time for measuring the outcomes. The theory defines clearly and specifically the variables to be studied; delineates the relationships among extraneous, treatment, and outcomes variables; and directs the statistical analyses. Therefore, it guides the interpretation of findings and improves the validity of conclusions. Furthermore, theory enhances the clinical relevance and applicability of the research findings. Clinicians are concerned with providing interventions to real-life clients, who differ from carefully selected research participants, in real-life situations, which differ from the controlled research conditions in that multiple factors influence outcomes achievement. Clinicians are held accountable for the care or treatment they give. Therefore, they should know not only that the treatment "works" (it produces the desired outcomes) but also why and how it works in order to prescribe the most appropriate intervention(s) to their clients. Clinicians who are aware of the why, what, how, when, where, and for whom of interventions are better informed when making care-related decisions (Goldfried & Wolfe, 1996).

To illustrate the advantages of the theory-driven approach to effectiveness research in enhancing the clinical relevance and applicability of the study findings, let us take the example of the psychoeducational interventions examined in the SHIP study. Two middle-range theories informed the design of the self-help and uncertainty management interventions. The interventions aimed at assisting women with breast cancer receiving adjuvant therapy in their adjustment to illness. A framework was developed to operationalize the intervention theories. The framework specified the relationships among extraneous, intervention, and outcomes variables (for a detailed description of the study, refer to Sidani, 1994). Extraneous variables included client personal characteristics (such as state anxiety) and health- and illness-related characteristics (such as stage of cancer), as well as resources available to clients (such as social support). The intervention variables included the component and dosage actually received by the participants. The intermediate outcomes variables mediating the intervention effects on the ultimate outcome were knowledge, uncertainty, affect, and self-care activities; the ultimate outcome was life quality. The direct and moderating effects of the extraneous and intervention variables on the outcomes variables were tested using individual regression analyses. The analyses were conducted on the subgroup of 56 women who remained over the six points of data collection (i.e., one year posttest). Only selected findings are presented here for illustration. Findings indicated (a) women who attended a large number of the six planned self-help classes demonstrated improvement in self-care abilities; (b) women who received a large number of the six planned phone contacts during which all their concerns were successfully addressed demonstrated reduced uncertainty; (c) educational background, sense of mastery, symptom extension, work status, size of social network, and use of available social support strengthened the effects of the interventions on knowledge, self-care ability, and negative affect; and (d) state anxiety weakened the effects of the interventions on knowledge and self-care ability. These results supported the theoretical propositions of the framework that operationalized the intervention theory.

   These findings have implications for clinicians planning to apply the self-help and uncertainty management interventions in their practice. The self-help classes are most effective (i.e., largest effect size) in enhancing self-care abilities. The uncertainty management intervention is most effective and efficient in reducing uncertainty. This implies that the interventions should be judiciously applied to induce changes in specific outcomes, as specified in the intervention theory. The interventions are distinct and specific and cannot be used interchangeably to achieve the same outcomes. Clinicians prescribing the self-help or the uncertainty management interventions should encourage their clients to attend all the scheduled intervention sessions in order to benefit most from the intervention. Also, clinicians should be aware that the two interventions are most helpful for women with high education, high sense of control over events (i.e., sense of mastery), full-time job, and a large social network, who use the available support and experience no or minimal worsening of their symptoms. Alternative interventions or modes of delivering the interventions could be designed to meet the needs of women with low education, low sense of mastery, restricted social support and worsening symptoms. The self-help and uncertainty management interventions are less useful for women experiencing high state anxiety, since this characteristic interfered with learning about self-care. Attempts to reduce the clients' anxiety could be initiated before starting the scheduled intervention sessions. The detailed information obtained in this theory-driven effectiveness study is clinically relevant as it guides clinicians in deciding who among their clients would benefit most from the interventions Further testing of these interventions is on-going..

Operationalizing the Theory-Driven Evaluation

The advantages gained from the application of the theory-driven approach to effectiveness research makes it a useful and appropriate methodology for clinical nursing research. The strategies for operationalizing this approach have been extensively discussed in the previous chapters. Here we summarize the implications for conducting effectiveness research in the real world.

Various research designs can be used to evaluate a particular intervention— that is, the choice of a research design cannot be made simply on the basis of rigor alone (Jacobson & Christensen, 1996; Rossi & Freeman, 1985). Pure experimental designs may not lend themselves to the study of complex situations in real-world field settings (Hegyvary, 1993). Experimental designs usually focus on maintaining the internal validity of a study, which is necessary for demonstrating the causal connection between the intervention and the outcomes, and they are based on the assumptions of initial equivalence, uniformity of treatment implementation, and uniformity of the subjects' response to treatment. In the field setting, multiple factors contribute to outcomes achievement. These factors interfere with the full participation by the target population, with the ability to control for extraneous factors, and with the ability to standardize the intervention activities and its delivery, resulting in differential subjects' response to the treatment and difficulty in interpreting the findings (Lipsey, Crosse, Dunkle, Pollard, & Stobart, 1985; Rossi, 1978). Therefore, the focus in field effectiveness research is *not* only on demonstrating the causal connection between the intervention and the outcomes but rather on understanding the processes underlying the intervention effects (i.e., causal explanation). Construct validity of a study is of prime concern when attempting to explain how and why the intervention effects are produced (Conrad & Conrad, 1994). Consequently, alternative design strategies are needed to test the effectiveness of interventions in the complexity of the real world. The alternative designs must allow for representing subjects' self-selection into the type and amount of treatment, examining the influence of extraneous factors on the treatment delivery and on outcomes, assessing the implementation of the intervention and the processes mediating the intervention effects, and determining the level of change expected in intermediate and ultimate outcomes. Correlational designs, such as surveys, naturalistic observational and regression-discontinuity designs, multiple case studies designs, and quasi-experimental designs, are examples of alternative design strategies. Careful operationalization of constructs and careful analysis of the influence of multiple factors represent the strengths of these types of designs in dealing with the different types of validity. Designs that combine elements of the conventional experimental and alternative designs are needed for a comprehensive, valid evaluation of interventions.

The timing for measuring the outcomes is another design issue that needs to be addressed when planning an effectiveness study. The simple pretest-posttest design can fall short of detecting the expected pattern of change in the outcomes, especially when the most pronounced changes are theoretically predicted to occur weeks or months after the intervention delivery. Therefore, repeated measurements of outcome variables after intervention delivery are crucial for capturing the expected pattern of change in the outcomes. Describing and examining the pattern of change in the outcomes is a useful indicator of the intervention effectiveness not only in producing the effect at a particular point in time but also in maintaining the desired changes over time, which is the ultimate goal of health-related interventions. Knowing the true pattern of change in outcomes informs clinicians of the treatment effectiveness, of when to conclude treatment, and of the necessity for changing the strength of the intervention to achieve the desired outcomes.

Understanding subjects' self-selection into treatment and into level of treatment is essential for identifying subgroups of the target population for whom the intervention is most appropriate and most effective. This kind of analysis requires careful follow-up of cases and inquiry about clients' reasons for entry or nonentry into treatment. Comparisons of subjects who refused to participate, who dropped out at different points in time, and who received different strengths of the intervention, on relevant personal and health-related characteristics, must be done. Results of these comparisons point to client characteristics that correlate with the intervention variables, thereby confounding its effects. Knowledge of reasons given for nonparticipation assists in identifying factors related to the clients, setting, intervener, and intervention that influence the clients' decision to enter treatment and consequently in providing for clues on what aspect of the situation can be improved to make treatment more attractive and appropriate to various clients. Attrition or dropping out of the experimental groups reduces the statistical power for detecting significant effects. It also threatens the external validity of conclusions, since it may be associated with various factors related to the participants or to the intervention that limit the applicability of the intervention to the target client population. Examples of factors leading to attrition include but are not limited to participants feeling that they are not benefiting from the intervention being evaluated, participants feeling that they have improved after receiving a particular dose of the intervention and that they do not need to continue the treatment (this factor has implications for determining the most effective dosage of the intervention), deterioration of the participants' health condition precluding them from continuing the intervention activities, participants' lack of satisfaction with or acceptance of some aspects of the intervention or its method of delivery or with the interaction with the intervener, participants' perception that the intervention does not meet their individual needs, and other personal factors (such as age, losing interest in the study, transportation problems). Knowledge of which factor(s) was (were) responsible for attrition expands our understanding of which aspect of the intervention is acceptable to which group of participants, of which minimal dosage is required for producing what level of change in the outcomes, and of how the intervention or its mode of delivery could be improved or refined to make it attractive and appropriate to various clients.

The actual intervention component(s) received by the participants, rather than group assignment, must be recorded; when the intervention or program is composed of different components that are delivered based on the individual needs of participants, the component(s) received by each participant should be documented. Analyzing the impact of each intervention component on the intended outcomes increases the specificity of the study findings; that is, these findings depict the differential effects of the intervention components on the intended outcomes, indicating which component is most effective in producing which outcome. This piece of information enhances the construct validity of the intervention and provides the basis for appropriate clinical decision making. Participants in the control group should be asked whether or not they received any component of the intervention or a similar intervention, in order to determine the extent to which the treatment was disseminated. Those who received some component of the intervention cannot be considered true controls. Leaving them in the control group and reduces the size of the contrast between the experimental and the control groups on the outcomes variable. Such persons could be added to the experimental group or included into a separate, experimental or placebo group.

In addition to recording the intervention component received by the participants, the actual strength of the intervention received by each participant is to be measured and used in the analysis as the predictor of mediating or outcomes variables (based on the propositions of the intervention theory). Including the strength of the intervention in the analyses, instead of the simple group membership variable (as is conventionally done in intention-to-treat analysis), has some advantages. It reduces the error of measurement in the independent variable (i.e., the intervention) and consequently the within-experimental group variance, thus increasing the statistical power for detecting significant effects; it also allows for determination of dose-response function, which is essential for prescribing the intervention dosage that is most effective in producing the outcomes. Methods for measuring the strength of a particular intervention may vary with its nature and are not yet well known. Efforts to develop tools to measure intervention strength are needed.

Clients' characteristics contributing to the intervention effects must be measured and their impact determined, whether the study design is experimental or nonexperimental. The particular characteristics to be measured and their direct, indirect, or conditioning effects to be tested are derived from the intervention theory. A causal modeling approach or subgroup analysis is used to analyze these effects. Determining the contribution of the clients' characteristics to the intervention effects provides a clear understanding of which client population would benefit most from the intervention, thus improving external validity of the findings and offering clinicians a sound knowledge base for prescribing the intervention appropriately.

Analyzing the contribution of the intervention component and dosage and the characteristics of clients, interveners, and settings to outcomes achievement involves examination of their direct and moderating effects on the outcomes variables. Such analyses entail conducting subgroup analyses or testing the theoretical model of these effects through path or structural equation modeling analyses. Both types of analyses incorporate numerous variables and require the use of sophisticated multivariate statistics. Therefore, the sample size needed to perform the analyses with adequate statistical power should be carefully determined through a power analysis.

Process evaluation is viewed as an essential aspect of effectiveness research, as it determines which factors related to the setting, the intervener, and the intervention delivery system facilitate or hinder the achievement of the intended outcomes. Results of process evaluation specify the conditions under which the intervention is most effective and inform future application of the intervention in various settings.

Careful selection of instruments measuring the variables of interest is important for ensuring construct validity. In particular, the sensitivity of outcomes measures needs to be assessed prior to data collection and during data analysis. Methods for evaluating the sensitivity of the measures to change (i.e., responsiveness) must be refined, however. Furthermore, the focus on and efforts for enhancing the validity of outcome measurement in effectiveness research should not detract from clinical relevance. Investigators should consider selecting clinically relevant outcomes, that is, those of interest to clinicians, clients, and policymakers yet reflective of the specific intervention effects, and using measures that are valid, yet applicable to the field setting, easy to administer, easy for clients to respond to (i.e., they should be relatively short yet comprehensive), and providing information that is interpretable and meaningful to clinicians and clients if the ultimate goal is the application of the intervention in everyday practice.

When guided by theory that explains presenting problems and the processes underlying the intervention given to resolve or manage the problem, intervention evaluation research contributes to the development of basic as well as applied or clinical knowledge (Hawkins, 1978). The theory-driven approach to effectiveness research not only attempts to determine the success of an intervention in producing the expected outcomes; it provides a medium for developing, testing, and refining descriptive and prescriptive theories that are needed to guide practice.

Determining the contribution to outcomes achievement of multiple factors related to client, setting, intervener, and intervention is a major undertaking. It may be accomplished in a large multisite effectiveness study, guided by theory and requiring complex planning, implementation, and analyses to capture all relevant extraneous, intervention, and outcomes variables. Or it can be accomplished through replication studies. A series of intervention evaluation studies are planned, where relevant factors (such as client subgroups, setting, dosage, intervener) are systematically varied to determine their unique contribution to outcomes. Studies have to progress from examining the impact of one factor to including multiple factors simultaneously.

In conclusion, theory-driven effectiveness research should not be guided by a single design or research method. Resorting to a single research method leads to findings that are constrained by the limitations and biases of the method used (Chen & Rossi, 1989). Rather, multiple and diverse research methods (including design, methods for data collection, and strategies for data analysis) are needed to enhance the validity of findings: Effectiveness research should be conducted within a critical multiplistic orientation (Cook, 1985).

REFERENCES

Adelman, H. S. (1986). Intervention theory and evaluating efficacy. *Evaluation Review, 10(1),* 65-83.

Altose, M., Cherniack, N., & Fishman, A. P. (1985). Respiratory sensations and dyspnea. *Journal of Applied Physiology, 58(4),* 1051-1054.

Archbold, P. G., Stewart, B. J., Miller, L. L., Harvath, T. A., Greenlick, M. R., Van Buren, L., Kirsechling, J. M., Valanis, B. G., Brody, K. K., Schook, J. E., & Hagan, J. M. (1995). The PREP system of nursing interventions: A pilot test with families caring for older members. *Research in Nursing and Health, 18,* 3-16.

Barlow, D. H. (1996). Health care policy, psychotherapy research, and the future of psychotherapy. *American Psychologist, 51(10),* 1050-1058.

Bauman, K. E., Viadro, C. I., & Tsui, A. O. (1994). Use of true experimental designs for family planning program evaluation: Merits, problems and solutions. *International Family Planning Perspectives, 20(3),* 108-113.

Basch, C. E., & Gold, R. S. (1986). The dubious effects of type V errors in hypothesis testing on health education practice and theory. *Health Education Research, 1(4),* 299-305.

Bejar, I. I. (1980). Biased assessment of program impact due to psychometric artifacts. *Psychological Bulletin, 87(3),* 513-524.

Bentler, P. M. (1992). *EQS program manual.* Los Angeles, CA: BMDP Statistical Software.

Beutler, L. E. (1991). Have all won and must all have prizes? Revisiting Luborsky et al.'s verdict. *Journal of Consulting and Clinical Psychology, 59(2),* 226-232.

Bickman, L. (1985). Improving established statewide programs. A component theory of evaluation. *Evaluation Review, 9(2),* 189-208.

Bittner, V., & Oberman, A. (1993). Efficacy studies in coronary rehabilitation. *Cardiology Clinics, 11(2),* 333-347.

Bloch, D. (1975). Evaluation of nursing care in terms of process and outcome: Issues in research and quality assurance. *Nursing Research, 24(4),* 256-263.

Bond, S., & Thomas, L. H. (1991). Issues in measuring outcomes of nursing. *Journal of Advanced Nursing, 16,* 1492-1502.

Bond, S., & Thomas, L. H. (1992). Input on outcomes. *Nursing Mirror, 16(88),* 50-52.

Boruch, R., & Gomez, H. (1977). Sensitivity, bias, and theory in impact evaluations. *Professional Psychology, 8,* 411-434.

Braden, C. J. (1990). Learned self-help response to chronic illness experience: A test of three alternative learning theories. *Scholarly Inquiry for Nursing Practice: An International Journal, 4(1),* 23-40.

Braden, C. J., Mishel, M. H., Longman, A., & Burns, L. R. (1989). *Nurse interventions promoting self-help response to breast cancer* (Grant No. NCI 1R01 CA48450-01A1). Washington, DC: National Cancer Institute.

Braden, C. J., Sidani, S., Ferketich, S., & Verran, J. (1993, September). *Instrumentation for intervention studies.* Workshop presented at the National Conference on Instrumentation, Tucson, AZ.

Brooten, D., & Naylor, M. D. (1995). Nurses' effect on changing patient outcomes. *Image: Journal of Nursing Scholarship, 27(2),* 95-99.

Brown, S. A. (1992). Meta-analysis of diabetes patient education research: Variations in intervention effects across studies. *Research in Nursing and Health, 15,* 409-419.

Bryk, A. S., & Raudenbush, S. W. (1992). *Hierarchical linear models: Applications and data analysis methods.* Newbury Park, CA: Sage.

Bulechek, G. M., & McCloskey, J. C. (1992). *Nursing interventions: Essential nursing treatments* (2nd ed.). Philadelphia: W. B. Saunders.

Burchinal, M., & Applebaum, M. I. (1991). Estimating individual development functions: Methods and their assumptions. *Child Development, 62,* 23-43.

Burns, N., & Grove, S. K. (1993). *The practice of nursing research. Conduct, critique and utilization* (2nd ed.). Philadelphia: W. B. Saunders.

Burrows-Hudson, S. (1995). Nephrology clinical outcomes: Part 1. Mortality, morbidity, adequacy of treatment, and quality of life. *ANNA Journal, 22(2),* 113-121.

Caldwell, J. R., Cobb, S., Dawling, M. D., & deJough, D. (1970). The dropout problem in antihypertensive treatment. *Journal of Chronic Disease, 22,* 579.

Campbell, A. (1981). *The sense of well-being in America. Recent patterns and trends.* New York: McGraw-Hill.

Campbell, A., Converse, P. E., & Rodgers, W. L. (1976). *The quality of American life.* New York: Russell Sage.

Candeias, N. M. F. (1991). Evaluating the quality of health education programmes. *Hygiene, 10(2),* 40-44.

Caplan, N. (1968). Treatment intervention and reciprocal interaction effects. *Journal of Social Issues, 24(1),* 63-88.

Carter, J. H., Moorhead, S. A., McCloskey, J. C., & Bulechek, G. M. (1995). Using the nursing interventions classification to implement agency for health care policy and research guidelines. *Journal of Nursing Care Quality, 9(2),* 76-86.

Caruso, C. C., Hadley, B. J., Shukla, R., Frame, P., & Khoury, J. (1992). Cooling effects and comfort of four cooling blanket temperatures in humans with fever. *Nursing Research, 41(2),* 68-72.

Carver, R. P. (1974). Two dimensions of tests: Psychometric and edumetric. *American Psychologist, 29,* 512-518.

Chen, H. T. (1989). The conceptual framework of the theory-driven perspective. *Evaluation and Program Planning, 12,* 391-396.

Chen, H. T. (1990). *Theory-driven evaluations.* Newbury Park, CA: Sage.

Chen, H. T. (1994). Current trends and future directions in program evaluation. *Evaluation Practice, 15(3),* 229-238.

Chen, H. T., & Rossi, P. H. (1980). The multi-goal, theory-driven approach to evaluation: A model linking basic and applied social science. *Social Forces, 59(1),* 107-122.

Chen, H. T., & Rossi, P. H. (1983). Evaluating with sense. The theory-driven approach. *Evaluation Review, 7(3),* 283-302.

Chen, H. T., & Rossi, P. H. (1987). The theory-driven approach to validity. *Evaluation and Program Planning, 10,* 95-103.

Chen, H. T., & Rossi, P. H. (1989). Issues in the theory-driven perspective. *Evaluation and Program Planning, 12,* 199-306.

Christman, N. J., McConnell, E. A., Pfieffer, C., Webster, K. K., Schmitt, M., & Ries, J. (1988). Uncertainty, coping, and distress following infarction: Transition from hospital to home. *Research in Nursing & Health, 11,* 71-82.

Close, P., Burkey, E., Kazak, A., Danz, P., & Lange, B. (1995). A prospective, controlled evaluation of home chemotherapy for children with cancer. *Pediatrics, 95(6),* 896-900.

Closs, S. J., & Tierney, A. J. (1993). The complexities of using a structure, process and outcome framework: The case of an evaluation of discharge planning for elderly patients. *Journal of Advanced Nursing, 18,* 1279-1287.

Cohen, P. (1982). To be or not to be. Control and balancing of type I and type II errors. *Evaluation and Program Planning, 5,* 247-253.

Condelli, W. S., & Hubbard, R. L. (1994). Relationship between time spent in treatment and client outcomes from therapeutic communities. *Journal of Substance Abuse Treatment, 11(1),* 25-33.

Conn, V. S., Taylor, S. G., & Casey, B. (1992). Cardiac rehabilitation program participation and outcomes after myocardial infarction. *Rehabilitation Nursing, 17(2),* 58-62.

Conrad, K. J., & Conrad, K. M. (1994). Reassessing validity threats in experiments: Focus on construct validity. *New Directions for Program Evaluation, 63,* 5-26.

Cook, T. (1985). Postpositivist critical multiplism. In R. Shotlans & M. Mark (Eds.), *Social science and social policy* (pp. 21-61). Beverly Hills, CA: Sage.

Cook, T. D. (1993). A quasi-sampling theory of the generalization of causal relationships. *New Directions for Program Evaluation, 57,* 39-82.

Cook, T. D., & Campbell, D. T. (1979). *Quasi-experimentation. Design and analysis issues for field settings.* Boston: Houghton Mifflin.

Cook, T. J., & Poole, W. K. (1982). Treatment implementation and statistical power. A research note. *Evaluation Review, 6(3),* 425-430.

Cooper, J., & Croyle, R. T. (1984). Attitudes and attitude change. *Annual Review of Psychology, 35,* 395-426.

Costner, H. L. (1989). The validity of conclusions in evaluation research: A further development of Chen and Rossi's theory-driven approach. *Evaluation and Program Planning, 12,* 345-353.

Crano, W. D., & Messe, L. A. (1985). Assessing and redressing comprehension artifacts in social intervention research. *Evaluation Review, 9(2),* 144-172.

Crits-Christoph, P., & Mintz, J. (1991). Implications of therapist effects for the design and analysis of comparative studies of psychotherapies. *Journal of Consulting and Clinical Psychology, 59(1),* 20-26.

Cronbach, L. J. (1992). *Designing evaluations of educational and social programs.* San Francisco: Jossey-Bass.

Cronbach, L. J., Gleser, G. C., Nanda, H., & Rajaratnam, N. (1972). *The dependability of behavioral measurements. Theory of generalizability of scores and profiles.* New York: John Wiley.

Daro, D., & McCurdy, K. (1994). Preventing child abuse and neglect: Programmatic interventions. *Child Welfare, 23(5),* 405-430.

Deal, L. W. (1994). The effectiveness of community health nursing interventions: A literature review. *Public Health Nursing, 11(5),* 315-323.

Deiriggi, P. M. (1990). Effects of waterbed flotation on indicators of energy expenditure in preterm infants. *Nursing Research, 39(3),* 140-147.

Deming, W. E. (1986). *Out of crisis.* Cambridge, MA: MIT, Center for Advanced Engineering Study.

Devine, E. C., O'Connor, F. W., Cook, T. D., Wenk, V. A., & Curtin, T. R. (1988). Clinical and financial effects of psychoeducational care provided by staff nurses to adult surgical patients in the post-DRG environment. *American Journal of Public Health, 78(10),* 1293-1297.

Devine, J. A., Wright, J. D., & Joyner, L. M. (1994). Issues in implementing a randomized experiment in a field setting. *New Directions for Program Evaluation, 63,* 27-40.

Deyo, R. A., & Centor, R. M. (1986). Assessing the responsiveness of functional scales to clinical change: An analogy to diagnostic test performance. *Journal of Chronic Disease, 39(11),* 897-906.

Deyo, R. A., & Inui, T. S. (1980). Dropouts and broken appointments. *Medical Care, 17,* 1146.

Deyo, R. A., & Inui, T. S. (1984). Toward clinical applications of health status measures: Sensitivity of scales to clinically important changes. *Health Services Research, 19(3),* 275-290.

Dignan, M. B., Michielutte, R., Sharp, P. C., Young, L. D., & Daniels, L. A. (1991). Use of process evaluation to guide health education in Forsyth county's project to prevent cervical cancer. *Public Health Reports, 106(1),* 73-77.

Donabedian, A. (1980). *The definition of quality and approaches to its assessment.* Ann Arbor, MI: Health Administration Press.

Donabedian, A. (1988). The quality of care: How can it be defined? *Journal of the American Medical Association, 260,* 1743-1748.

Donabedian, A., Wheeler, J. R. C., & Wyszewianski, L. (1982). Quality, cost, and health: An integrative model. *Medical Care, 20,* 975-992.

Donner, A. (1992). Randomized trials for assessing interventions in primary care: Discussion. In F. Tudiver, M. J. Bass, E. V. Dunn, P. G. Norton, & M. Stewart (Eds.), *Assessing interventions. Traditional and innovative methods* (pp. 62-67). Newbury Park, CA: Sage.

Droitcour, J. A., & Chelimsky, E. (1995, November). *Cross design synthesis: Concept, method, and application.* Paper presented at the American Evaluation Association Conference, Vancouver, B.C.

Duryee, R. (1992). The efficacy of inpatient education after myocardial infarction. *Heart & Lung, 21(3),* 217-227.

Einhorn, H. J., & Hogarth, R. M. (1986). Judging probable cause. *Psychological Bulletin, 99(1),* 3-19.

Eisenhauer, L. A. (1994). A typology of nursing therapeutics. *Image: Journal of Nursing Scholarship, 26(4),* 261-264.

Ellwood, P. M. (1988). A technology of patient experience: The Shattuck lecture—outcomes management. *New England Journal of Medicine, 318(23),* 1549-1556.

Epstein, D. (1995). Characteristics of the intervener. *Proceedings of the Western Institute of Nursing-Research Conference, 28,* 316.

Erben, R., Franzkowiak, P., & Wenzel, E. (1992). Assessment of the outcomes of health intervention. *Social Science and Medicine, 35(4),* 359-365.

Finnerty, F. A., Mattie, E. C., & Finnerty, F. A. (1973). Hypertension in the inner city: 1. Analysis of clinical dropouts. *Circulation, 47*, 73.

Finney, J. W., & Moos, R. H. (1984). Environmental assessment and evaluation research: Examples from mental health and substance abuse programs. *Evaluation and Program Planning, 7*, 151-167.

Finney, J. W., & Moos, R. H. (1989). Theory and method in treatment evaluation. *Evaluation and Program Planning, 12*, 307-316.

Francis, D. J., Fletcher, J. M., Stuebing, K. K., Davidson, K. C., & Thompson, N. M. (1991). Analysis of change. Modeling individual growth. *Journal of Consulting and Clinical Psychology, 39(1)*, 27-37.

Frank-Stomborg, M., Pender, N. J., Walker, S. N., & Sechrist, K. R. (1990). Determinants of health-promoting lifestyle in ambulatory cancer patients. *Social Science and Medicine, 31*, 1159-1168.

French, M. T. (1995). Economic evaluation of drug abuse treatment programs: Methodology and findings. *American Journal of Drug and Alcohol Abuse, 21*(1), 111-135.

Gallagher-Thompson, D., & Steffen, A. M. (1994). Comparative effects of cognitive-behavioral and brief psychodynamic psychotherapies for depressed family caregivers. *Journal of Consulting and Clinical Psychology, 62(3)*, 543-549.

Gierszewski, S. (1983). The relationship of weight loss, locus of control and social support. *Nursing Research, 32*, 43-47.

Glass, G. V., McGaw, B., & Smith, M. (1981). *Meta-analysis in social research.* Beverly Hills, CA: Sage.

Goldfried, M. R., & Wolfe, B. E. (1996). Psychotherapy practice and research. Repairing a strained alliance. *American Psychologist, 51(10)*, 1007-1016.

Gottfried, S. B., Altose, M. D., Kelson, S. G., & Cherniack, N. S. (1981). Perception of changes in airflow resistance in obstructive pulmonary disorders. *American Review of Respiratory Diseases, 124*, 566-570.

Green, L. W., & Lewis, F. M. (1986). *Measurement and evaluation in health education and health promotion.* Palo Alto, CA: Mayfield.

Griffiths, P. (1995). Progress in measuring nursing outcomes. *Journal of Advanced Nursing, 21*, 1092-1100.

Guyatt, G. H., Deyo, R. A., Charlson, M., Levine, M. N., & Mitchell, A. (1989). Responsiveness and validity in health status measurement: A clarification. *Journal of Clinical Epidemiology, 42(5)*, 403-408.

Guyatt, G. H., Feeny, D. H., & Patrick, D. L. (1993). Measuring health-related quality of life. *Annals of Internal Medicine, 118*, 622-629.

Guyatt, G. H., Kirshner, B., & Jaeschke, R. (1992). Measuring health status: What are the necessary measurement properties. *Journal of Clinical Epidemiology, 45(12)*, 1341-1345.

Halverson, H. W., Cohen, S. J., Brekke, K. L., McClatchey, M. W., & Cohen, M. M. (1993). Process evaluation of a system (partners for prevention) for prevention-oriented primary care. *Evaluation and the Health Professions, 16(1)*, 96-105.

Hawkes, J. M., & Holm, K. (1993). Gender differences in exercise determinants. *Nursing Research, 42(3)*, 166- 172.

Hawkins, D. F. (1978). Applied research and social theory. *Evaluation Quarterly, 2(1)*, 141-152.

Hegyvary, S. T. (1991). Issues in outcomes research. *Journal of Quality Assurance, 5(2)*, 1-6.

Hegyvary, S. T. (1993). Patient care outcomes related to management of symptoms. *Annual Review of Nursing Research, 11,* 145-168.

Hegyvary, S. T., & Chamings, P. A. (1975). The hospital setting and patient care outcomes. *Journal of Nursing Administration, 5(4),* 36-42.

Heller, K. (1990). Social and community intervention. *Annual Review of Psychology, 41,* 141-168.

Hoefer, R. (1994). A good story, well told: Rules for evaluating human services programs. *Social Work, 39(2),* 233-236.

Hollon, S. D. (1996). The efficacy and effectiveness of psychotherapy relative to medications. *American Psychologist, 51(10),* 1025-1030.

Howard, K. I., Kopta, S. M., Krause, M. S., & Orlinsky, D. E. (1986). The dose-effect relationship in psychotherapy. *American Psychologist, 41(2),* 159-164.

Howard, K. I., Moras, K., Brill, P. L., Martinovich, Z., & Lutz, W. (1996). Efficacy, effectiveness, and patient progress. *American Psychologist, 51*(10), 1059-1064.

Hoyle, R. H. (Ed.). (1995). *Structural equation modeling: Concepts, issues, and applications.* Thousand Oaks, CA: Sage.

Inzer, F., & Aspinal, M. J. (1981). Evaluating patient outcomes. *Nursing Outlook, 29,* 178-181.

Jacobson, N. S., & Christensen, A. (1996). Studying the effectiveness of psychotherapy. How well can clinical trials do the job? *American Psychologist, 51(10),* 1031-1039.

Jacobson, N. S., & Truax, P. (1991). Clinical significance: A statistical approach to defining meaningful change in psychotherapy research. *Journal of Consulting and Clinical Psychology, 59(1),* 12-19.

Jennings, B. M. (1991). Patient outcomes research: Seizing the opportunity. *Advances in Nursing Science, 14(2),* 59-72.

Johnson, J. L., Ratner, P. A., Bottroff, J. L., & Hayduk, L. A. (1993). An exploration of Pender's health promotion model using LISREL. *Nursing Research, 42(3),* 132-138.

Jones, K. R. (1993). Outcomes analysis: Methods and issues. *Nursing Economics, 11(3),* 145-152.

Judd, C. M., & Kenny, D. A. (1981). Process analysis. Estimating mediation in treatment evaluations. *Evaluation Review, 5(5),* 602-619.

Keppel, G. (1991). *Design and analysis. A researcher's handbook* (3rd ed.). Englewood Cliffs, NJ: Prentice Hall.

King, J. A., Morris, L. L., & Fitz-Gibbon, C. T. (1987). *How to assess program implementation.* Newbury Park, CA: Sage.

Kirchhoff K. T., & Dille C.A. 1994. Issues in intervention research: Maintaining integrity. *Applied Nursing Research, 7(1),* 32-46.

Kirshner, B., & Guyatt, G. (1985). A methodological framework for assessing health indices. *Journal of Chronic Disease, 38(1),* 27-36.

Kotwall, C. A., Mahoney, L. J., Myers, R. E., & Decoste, L. (1992). Reasons for non-entry in randomized clinical trials for breast cancer: A single institutional study. *Journal of Surgical Oncology, 50,* 125-129.

Kremer, B. K. (1991). Physician recertification and outcomes assessment. *Evaluation and the Health Professions, 14(2),* 187-200.

Lam, J. A., Hartwell, S. W., & Jekel, J. F. (1994). "I prayed real hard, so I know I'll get in": Living with randomization. *New Directions for Program Evaluation, 63,* 55-66.

Lang, N. M., & Marek, K. D. (1990). The classification of patient outcomes. *Journal of Professional Nursing, 6(3),* 158-163.

Lang, N. M., & Marek, K. D. (1991, November). *Clinical conditions and interventions: Their relationship to outcomes: Outcomes that reflect clinical practice.* Paper presented at Patient Outcome Research: Examining the Effectiveness of Nursing Practice, National Center for Nursing Research, Rockville, MD.

Larrabee, J. H. (1996). Emerging model of quality. *Image: Journal of Nursing Scholarship, 28(4),* 353-358.

LeFort, S. (1993). The statistical versus clinical significance debate. *Image: Journal of Nursing Scholarship, 25(1),* 57-62.

Lipsey, M. W. (1990). *Design sensitivity: Statistical power for experimental research.* Newbury Park, CA: Sage.

Lipsey, M. W. (1993). Theory as method: Small theories of treatments. *New Directions for Program Evaluation, 57,* 5-38.

Lipsey, M. W., Crosse, S., Dunkle, J., Pollard, J., & Stobart, G. (1985). Evaluation: The state of the art and the sorry state of the science. *New Directions for Program Evaluation, 27,* 7-28.

Lipsey, M. W., & Pollard, J. A. (1989). Driving toward theory in program evaluation: More models to choose from. *Evaluation and Program Planning, 12,* 317-328.

Lohr, K. N. (1988). Outcome measurement: Concepts and questions. *Inquiry, 25,* 37-50.

Lowery, B. J., & DuCette, S. (1976). Disease-related learning and disease control in diabetes as a function of locus of control. *Nursing Research, 25,* 358-362.

Lundeman, B., Asplund, K., & Norbeg, A. (1990). Living with diabetes: Perceptions of well-being. *Research in Nursing and Health, 13,* 255-262.

Maas, M. L., Johnson, M., & Moorhead, S. (1996). Classifying nursing-sensitive outcomes. *Image: Journal of Nursing Scholarship, 28(4),* 295-301.

Malec, J. F., Smigielski, J. S., & DePompolo, R. W. (1991). Goal attainment scaling and outcome measurement in postacute brain injury rehabilitation. *Archives of Physical Medicine and Rehabilitation, 72,* 138-143.

Marfo, K., & Dinero, T. E. (1993). Assessing early intervention outcomes—Beyond program variables. *International Journal of Disability, Development and Education, 38(3),* 289-303.

Mariner, W. K. (1994). Outcomes assessment in health care reform: Promise and limitations. *American Journal of Law and Medicine, 10(1&2),* 37-57.

Mark, B. A. (1995). Patient outcomes research—A black box? *Image: Journal of Nursing Scholarship, 27(1),* 42.

Mark, M. M. (1983). Treatment implementation, statistical power, and internal validity. *Evaluation Review, 7(4),* 543-549.

Martin, K. S., & Scheet, N. J. (1992). *The Omaha system: Applications for community health nursing.* Philadelphia: W. B. Saunders.

Maxwell, S. E., & Delaney, H. D. (1993). Bivariate median split and spurious statistical significance. *Psychological Bulletin, 113(1),* 181-190.

McBride, S., Graydon, J., & Sidani, S. (1996). Dyspnea and anxiety in patients with COPD: The potential role of music. Unpublished manuscript.

McCloskey, J. C., Bulecheck, G. M., Cohen, M. Z., Craft, M. J., Crossley, J. D., Denehy, J. A., Glick, O. J., Kruckeberg, T., Maas, M., Prophet, C. M., & Tripp-Reimer, T. (1990). Classification of nursing intervention. *Journal of Professional Nursing, 6(3),* 151-157.

McHenry, J., Allen, C., Mishel, M. H., & Braden, C. J. (1993). Uncertainty management for women receiving treatment for breast cancer. In S. G. Funk, E. M. Tornquist, M. T. Champagne, & R. A. Wiese (Eds.), *Key aspects of caring for the chronically ill—hospital and home* (pp. 170-177). New York: Springer.

McNeely, E. A., & Clements, S. D. (1994). Recruitment and retention of the older adult into research studies. *Journal of Neuroscience Nursing, 26(1),* 57-61.

Meisenhelder, J. B. (1987). Anxiety: A block to clinical learning. *Nurse Educator, 12(6),* 27-30.

Messick, S. (1995). Validity of psychological assessment. *American Psychologist, 50(9),* 741-749.

Miller, P., Wikoff, R., Garrett, M. J., McMahon, M., & Smith, T. (1990). Regimen compliance two years after myocardial infarction. *Nursing Research, 36(6),* 333-336.

Mishel, M. H. (1988). Uncertainty in illness. *Image: Journal of Nursing Scholarship, 20(4),* 225-232.

Mishel, M. H. (1990). Reconceptualization of the uncertainty in illness theory. *Image: Journal of Nursing Scholarship, 22(4),* 256-262.

Mishel, M. H., & Braden, C. J. (1988). Finding meaning: Antecedents of uncertainty in women receiving treatment for gynecological cancer. *Nursing Research, 37(2),* 38-103.

Mitchell, P. H. (1993). Perspectives on outcome-oriented care systems. *Nursing Administration, 17(3),* 1-7.

Moritz, P. (1995, May). *Outcomes research: Examining clinical effectiveness.* Paper presented at the Western Institute of Nursing Conference, San Diego, CA.

Morse, E. V., Simon, P. M., Besch, C. L., & Walker, J. (1995). Issues of recruitment, retention, and compliance in community-based clinical trials with traditionally underserved populations. *Applied Nursing Research, 8(1),* 8-14.

Moskowitz, J. M. (1993). Why reports of outcome evaluations are often biased or uninterpretable. Examples from evaluations of drug abuse prevention programs. *Evaluation and Program Planning, 16,* 1-9.

Mullen, P. D., Mains, D. A., & Velez, R. (1992). A meta-analysis of controlled trials of cardiac patient education. *Patient Education and Counseling, 19,* 143-162.

Mumford, E., Schleisinger, H. J., & Glass, G. V. (1982). The effects of psychological intervention on recovery from surgery and heart attacks: An analysis of the literature. *American Journal of Public Health, 72(2),* 141-151.

Munro, B H., & Page, E. B. (1993). *Statistical methods for health care research* (2nd ed.). Philadelphia: J. B. Lippincott.

Nesselroade, J. R. (1991). Interindividual differences in intraindividual change. In L. M. Collins & J. L. Horn (Eds.), *Best methods for the analysis of change. Recent advances, unanswered questions, future directions* (pp. 92-105). Washington, DC: American Psychological Association.

Newman, F. L., & Tejeda, M. J. (1996). The need for research that is designed to support decisions in the delivery of mental health services. *American Psychologist, 51(10),* 1040-1049.

Nicewander, W. A., & Price, J. M. (1983). Reliability of measurement and the power of statistical tests: Some new results. *Psychological Bulletin, 94(3),* 524-533.

Oldridge, N. B., Guyatt, G. H, Fisher, M. E., & Rimm, A. A. (1988). Cardiac rehabilitation after myocardial infarction. Combined experience of randomized clinical trials. *Journal of the American Medical Association, 260(7),* 945-950.

Orwin, R. G., Cordray, D. S., & Huebner, R. B. (1994). Judicious application of randomized designs. *New Directions for Program Evaluation, 63,* 73-86.

Parker, S. O. (1983). A conceptual model for outcome assessment. *Nurse Practitioner, 8,* 44-45.

Payne, S. A. (1992). A study of life in cancer patients receiving palliative chemotherapy. *Social Science and Medicine, 35(12),* 1505-1509.

Pauley, P. A., & Cohen, S. (1984). Facilitating data-based decision-making. Manager's use of data in a community mental health center. *Evaluation Review, 8(2),* 205-224.

178   EVALUATING NURSING INTERVENTIONS

Peters, D. A. (1988). An overview of current research relating to long-term outcomes. *Nursing and Health Care, 10(3),* 133-136.

Pletsch, P. K., Howe, C., & Tenney, M. (1995). Recruitment of minority subjects for intervention research. *Image: Journal of Nursing Scholarship, 27(3),* 211-215.

Prochaska, J. O., DiClemente, C. C., & Norcross, J. C. (1992). In search of how people change: Applications to addictive behaviors. *American Psychologist, 47,* 1102-1114.

Raskin, I. E., & Maklan, C. W. (1991). Medical treatment effectiveness research: A view from inside the Agency for Health Care Policy and Research. *Evaluation and the Health Professions, 14(2),* 161-186.

Redfern, S. J., & Norman, I. J. (1990). Measuring the quality of nursing care: A consideration of different approaches. *Journal of Advanced Nursing, 15,* 1260-1271.

Reichardt, C. S. (1979). The statistical analysis of data from non-equivalent group designs. In T. D. Cook & D. T. Campbell (Eds.), *Quasi-experimentation: Design and analysis issues for field settings* (pp. 147-205). Skokie, IL: Rand McNally.

Reid, W. J., & Hanrahan, P. (1988). Measuring implementation of social treatment. *New Directions for Program Evaluation, 40,* 93-111.

Renfroe, K. L. (1988). Effect of progressive relaxation on dyspnea and state anxiety in patients with chronic obstructive pulmonary disease. *Heart & Lung, 17(4),* 408-413.

Rezmovic, E. L. (1984). Assessing treatment implementation amid the slings and arrows of reality. *Evaluation Review, 8(2),* 187-204.

Ribisl, K. M., Walton, M. A., Mowbray, C. T., Luke, D. A., Davidson, W. S. & Bootsmiller, B. J. (1996). Minimizing participant attrition in panel studies through the use of effective retention and tracking strategies: Review and recommendations. *Evaluation and Program Planning, 19(1),* 1-25.

Rice, V. H., & Johnson, J. E. (1984). Preadmission self-instruction booklets, preadmission exercise performance, and teaching time. *Nursing Research, 33(3),* 147-151.

Rogosa, D., Brandt, D., & Zimowski, M. (1982). A growth curve approach to measurement of change. *Psychological Bulletin, 92(3),* 726-748.

Rogosa, D. R., & Willet, J. B. (1985). Understanding correlates of change by modeling individual differences in growth. *Psychometrika, 50(2),* 203-228.

Rosen, A., & Proctor, E. K. (1978). Specifying the treatment process: The basis for effectiveness research. *Journal of Social Service Research, 2(1),* 25-43.

Rossi, P. H. (1978). Issues in the evaluation of human services delivery. *Evaluation Quarterly, 2(4),* 573-599.

Rossi, P. H., & Freeman, H. E. (1985). *Evaluation: A systematic approach* (3rd ed.). Beverly Hills, CA: Sage.

Rossi, P. H., & Freeman, H. E. (1993). *Evaluation: A systematic approach* (5th ed.). Newbury Park, CA: Sage.

Rossi, P. H., & Wright, J. D. (1984). Evaluation research: An assessment. *Annual Review of Sociology, 10,* 331-352.

Rubin, D. B. (1974). Estimating causal effects of treatments in randomized and nonrandomized studies. *Journal of Educational Psychology, 66(5),* 688-701.

Russell, D. W., & Buckwalter, K. C. (1991). Researching and evaluating model geriatric mental health programs: Part 2. Measurement of outcomes. *Archives of Psychiatric Nursing, 5(2),* 76-83.

Scheinder, A. L., & Darcy, R. E. (1984). Policy implications of using significance tests in evaluation research. *Evaluation Review, 8(4),* 573-582.

Scheirer, M. A., & Rezmovic, E. L. (1983). Measuring the degree of program implementation. A methodological review. *Evaluation Review, 7(5),* 599-633.

Schumacher, J. E., Milby, J. B., Raczynski, J. M., Engle, M., Caldwell, E. S., & Carr, J. A. (1994). Demoralization and threats to validity in Birmingham's homeless project. *New Directions for Program Evaluation, 63,* 41-44.

Schwartz, C. E., & Fox, B. H. (1995). Who says yes? Identifying selection biases in a psychosocial intervention study of multiple sclerosis. *Social Science and Medicine, 40(3),* 359-370.

Scott, A. G., & Sechrest, L. (1989). Strength of theory and theory of strength. *Evaluation and Program Planning, 12,* 329-336.

Sechrest, L. (1986). Modes and methods of personality research. *Journal of Personality, 54(1),* 318-331.

Sechrest, L., Ametrano, D., & Ametrano, I. M. (1983). Evaluations of social programs. In C. E. Walker (Ed.), *The handbook of clinical psychology* (pp. 129-166). Homewood, IL: Dow Jones-Irwin.

Seligman, M. E. P. (1996). Science as an ally to practice. *American Psychologist, 51(10),* 1072-1079.

Shadish, W. R., Cook, T. D., & Leviton, L. C. (1991). *Foundations of program evaluation: Theories of practice.* Newbury Park, CA: Sage.

Shapiro, J. Z. (1984). The social costs of methodological rigor: A note on the problem of massive attrition. *Evaluation Review, 8,* 705-712.

Shavelson, R. J., & Webb, N. M. (1991). *Generalizability theory: A primer.* Newbury Park, CA: Sage.

Shavelson, R. J., Webb, N. M., & Rowley, G. L. (1989). Generalizability theory. *American Psychologist, 44(6),* 922-932.

Shonkoff, J. P., Hause-Cramm, P., Krauss, M. W., & Upshur, C. C. (1988). Early intervention efficacy research: What have we learned and where do we go from here? *TEVSE, 8(1),* 81-93.

Sidani, S. (1991). *Effects of sedative music on the respiratory status of clients with COAD.* Unpublished master's thesis, University of Arizona, Tucson.

Sidani, S. (1994). *Empirical testing of a conceptual model to evaluate psychoeducational interventions.* Unpublished doctoral dissertation, University of Arizona, Tucson.

Siderovski, D. P., & Siderovski, S. L. (1992). Evaluating program effectiveness in health education research. *Canadian Journal of Program Evaluation, 7(2),* 43-60.

Simmons-Morton, D. G., Mullen, P. D., Mains, D. A., Tabak, E. R., & Green, L. W. (1992). Characteristics of controlled studies of patient education and counseling for preventive health behaviors. *Patient Education and Counseling, 19,* 175-204.

Slater, C. H. (1991). Outcomes assessment and management. *Evaluation and the Health Professions, 14(2),* 131-137.

Snyder, M., Egan, E. C., & Najima, Y. (1996). Defining nursing interventions. *Image: Journal of Nursing Scholarship, 28(2),* 137-142.

Soibelman, D. (1948). *Therapeutic and industrial uses of music: A review of the literature.* New York: Columbia University Press.

Steckler, A., Eng, E., & Goodman, R. M. (1991). Integrating qualitative and quantitative evaluation methods. *Hygie, 10(2),* 16-20.

Stevens, S. J. (1994). Common implementation issues in three large-scale social experiments. *New Directions for Program Evaluation, 63,* 45-54.

Stewart, B. J., & Archbold, P. G. (1992). Nursing interventions studies require outcome measures that are sensitive to change: Part 1. *Research in Nursing and Health, 15,* 477-481.

Stewart, B. J., & Archbold, P. G. (1993). Nursing interventions studies require outcome measures that are sensitive to change: Part 2. *Research in Nursing and Health, 16,* 77-81.

Strauss, A., & Corbin, J. (1994). Grounded theory methodology. An overview. In N. K. Denzin & Y. S. Lincoln (Eds.), *Handbook of qualitative research* (pp. 273-283). Thousand Oaks, CA: Sage.

Strupp, H. H. (1996). The tripartite model and the consumer reports study. *American Psychologist, 51(10),* 1017-1024.

Stucliffe, J. P. (1980). On the relationship of reliability to statistical power. *Psychological Bulletin, 88(2),* 509-515.

Tarlov, A. R., Ware, J. E., Greenfield, S., Nelson, E. C., Perrin, E., & Zubkoff, M. (1989). The medical outcomes study. An application of methods for monitoring the results of medical care. *Journal of the American Medical Association, 262(7),* 925-930.

Taylor, J. W. (1974). Measuring the outcomes of nursing care. *Nursing Clinics of North America, 9(2),* 337-348.

Thackwray, D. E., Smith, M. C., Bodfish, J. W., & Meyers, A. W. (1993). A comparison of behavioral and cognitive-behavioral interventions for bulimia nervosa. *Journal of Consulting and Clinical Psychology, 61(4),* 639-645.

Trochim, W. N. K. (1985). Pattern matching, validity, and conceptualization in program evaluation. *Evaluation Review, 9(5),* 575-604.

Walker, L. O., & Avant, K. C. (1989). *Strategies for theory construction in nursing* (2nd ed.). Norwalk, CT: Appleton & Lange.

Waltz, C. F., Strickland, O. L., & Lenz, E. R. (1991). *Measurement in nursing research* (2nd ed.). Philadelphia: F. A. Davis.

Wanich, C. K., Sullivan-Marx, E. M., Gottlieb, G. L., & Johnson, J. C. (1992). Functional status outcomes of a nursing intervention in hospitalized elderly. *Image: Journal of Nursing Scholarship, 24(3),* 201-207.

Warnecke, R. B., Flay, B. R., Kviz, F. J., Gruder, C. L., Langenberg, P., Crittenden, K. S., Mermelstein, R. J., Aitken, M., Wong, S. C., & Cook, T. D. (1991). Characteristics of participants in a televised smoking cessation intervention. *Preventive Medicine, 20,* 389-403.

Wildt, A R., & Ahtola, O. T. (1978). *Analysis of covariance.* Beverly Hills, CA: Sage.

Williams, J. I., & Naylor, D. (1992). How should health status measures be assessed? Cautionary notes on procrustean frameworks. *Journal of Clinical Epidemiology, 45(12),* 1347-1351.

Wong, C. A., & Bramwell, L. (1992). Uncertainty and anxiety after mastectomy for breast cancer. *Cancer Nursing, 15(5),* 363-371.

Yates, B. C. (1995). The relationships among social support and short- and long-term recovery outcomes in men with coronary heart disease. *Research in Nursing and Health, 18,* 193-203.

Yeaton, W. H. (1985). Using measures of treatment strength and integrity in planning research. *New Directions for Program Evaluation, 27,* 49-62.

Yeaton, W. H., & Sechrest, L. (1981). Critical dimensions in the choice and maintenance of successful treatments: Strength, integrity, and effectiveness. *Journal of Consulting and Clinical Psychology, 49(2),* 156-167.

Zeller, R. A., & Carmines, E. G. (1980). *Measurement in the social sciences.* Cambridge, UK: Cambridge University Press.

Zinn, J. S., Aaronson, W. E., & Rosko, M. D. (1993). Variations in the outcomes of care provided in Pennsylvania nursing homes. Facility and environmental correlates. *Medical Care, 31(6),* 475-487.

INDEX

ABOUT THE AUTHORS

Souraya Sidani, PhD, RN, is Assistant Professor at the Faculty of Nursing, University of Toronto. She teaches courses related to research methods and instrumentation. She consults with researchers and clinicians about issues related to the design and implementation of research projects and to the analysis of data. Her research areas of interest focus on evaluating health-related interventions and refining research methods and health-related measures for determining the clinical effectiveness of interventions. She developed and tested a conceptual framework for evaluating interventions, which formed the basis for this book. She has been involved in projects evaluating various interventions (such as the use of sedative music to relieve dyspnea in COPD patients, exercise to assist women with breast cancer in managing fatigue, and the use of an abilities-focused program of morning care in elderly with dementia), nursing care delivery models (such as the introduction of a collaborative care model), and educational programs (such as the primary care nurse practitioner program), with the primary responsibility of designing the evaluation study, managing data collection and entry, and conducting the statistical analyses. The topics of her publications relate to methodological issues, such as the comparison of quantitative and qualitative research methods, the comparison between repeated measures analysis of variance and individual regression analysis, the use of case studies in evaluation research, the application of the multitrait-multimethod logic for examining family relational data, and a discussion of methodological issues in assessing outcomes of care.

Carrie Jo Braden, PhD, RN, FAAN, is Associate Professor at the College of Nursing, University of Arizona. She teaches courses related to the development of middle-range theories and evaluation in nursing. She developed and tested the middle-range nursing theory of learned response to chronic illness experience. She also developed and evaluated a self-help intervention for patients with systemic lupus erythematosus and for women with breast cancer. Her research areas of interest include further testing of the learned response to chronic illness middle-range theory and evaluation of self-help interventions. The topics of her publications relate to the description and testing of the learned response to chronic illness theory and the evaluation of testing the effectiveness of the self-help interventions.